AN ETHICS CASEBOOK
FOR HOSPITALS

AN ETHICS CASEBOOK FOR HOSPITALS

PRACTICAL APPROACHES TO EVERYDAY ETHICS CONSULTATIONS

Second Edition

MARK G. KUCZEWSKI
ROSA LYNN B. PINKUS
KATHERINE WASSON

Georgetown University Press
Washington, DC

The publisher is not responsible for third-party websites or their content. URL links were active at time of publication.

Library of Congress Cataloging-in-Publication Data
Names: Kuczewski, Mark G., author. | Pinkus, Rosa Lynn B., author. |
    Wasson, Katherine, author.
Title: An Ethics Casebook for Hospitals : Practical Approaches to Everyday
    Ethics Consultations / Mark G. Kuczewski, Rosa Lynn B. Pinkus,
    Katherine Wasson.
Description: Second edition. | Washington, DC : Georgetown University
    Press, [2018] | Includes bibliographical references and index.
Identifiers: LCCN 2017028513 (print) | LCCN 2017031521 (ebook) | ISBN
    9781626165496 (hardcover : alk. paper) | ISBN 9781626165502 (pbk. : alk.
    paper) | ISBN 9781626165519 (ebook)
Subjects: LCSH: Medical ethics—Case studies. | Hospital care—Moral and
    ethical aspects—Case studies. | Medical ethics committees.
Classification: LCC R725.5 (ebook) | LCC R725.5 .K83 2018 (print) | DDC
    174.2—dc23
LC record available at https://lccn.loc.gov/2017028513

♾ This book is printed on acid-free paper meeting the requirements
of the American National Standard for Permanence in Paper for Printed
Library Materials.

18 17   9 8 7 6 5 4 3 2   First printing

Printed in the United States of America

Contents

Contents

SECTION II:
END-OF-LIFE DECISION MAKING

SECTION III:
DECISION MAKING FOR MINORS

Contents

Contents

Preface

When we consider how the health care landscape and clinical ethics have changed since the publication of the book's first edition, perhaps the old saying "The more things change, the more they stay the same" is apt. Much has, indeed, changed. But these changes are clearly recognizable and are developments built on the foundation laid in the 1990s.

The first edition of this book was developed from cases submitted by staff members of hospitals in the Consortium Ethics Program, the clinical ethics education network of western Pennsylvania that is centered at the University of Pittsburgh. It was founded and directed by one of the authors (Rosa Lynn B. Pinkus), and the cases were submitted as part of a training exercise. The exercise was meant to assist the participants in the program in developing their ability to analyze and respond to clinical ethics issues in their hospital. These participants, drawn from a wide variety of backgrounds and roles—including physicians, nurses, chaplains, and administrators—aimed to be ethics resource persons for their colleagues, even if they did not fully embrace the model of on-call clinical ethics consultation, which was a fairly new endeavor at the time. This second edition retains this guiding ideal of training frontline personnel to be ethics resources for their colleagues. However, the focus of this edition is *the development of the knowledge, skills, and attitudes needed to provide clinical ethics case consultations.*

This concept and practice of clinical ethics case consultation has certainly made much progress between editions. Although there is not at this writing a certification process for clinical ethics consultants, the American Society for Bioethics and Humanities (ASBH) has facilitated reaching a consensus on the core competencies that such professionals need to possess (American Society for Bioethics and Humanities 2011). An ASBH expert panel successfully piloted a portfolio assessment process that showed it is possible to assess the competencies of individual consultants with a reasonable amount of interrater reliability (Fins et al. 2013, 2016). This book (and its accompanying online materials) can be used by persons at any level of familiarity with clinical ethics, including students taking their first clinical ethics course, the hospital ethics committee member in need of formal training to supplement their experiential knowledge, and the professional who performs clinical ethics case consultations and wishes to sharpen and demonstrate their knowledge and skills. Below, we say more about the features of this book that will be of help.

This second edition contains twenty-six cases, thirteen that were carried over from the first edition and thirteen that are presented for the first time. Just as with the thirteen original cases, the thirteen new cases were encountered and reported on by health care professionals and administrators, sometimes through a formal clinical ethics consultation. Appropriate steps have been taken to alter the cases in order to meet standards for preserving patient confidentiality. The same guiding ideal was used to select the new cases as was used in the first edition. All the cases are relatively common scenarios, albeit particularized instances that could be encountered in almost any hospital or health system in the United States. No effort was made to include esoteric issues that seldom rise despite any theoretical interest such cases might generate. As a result, issues of informed consent, determination of the decision-making capacity of the patient to give consent or an informed refusal, and issues related to end-of-life decision making again dominate the content. Of course, the framework for making medical decisions for and with minors differs significantly from that for adults and requires its own section in order to appropriately address many similar treatment decisions.

All the cases in the organizational ethics section are new. These particular cases reflect the current national trends in underserved and marginalized patients, including undocumented immigrants, persons with substance use disorders, patients encountered during medical mission trips, and patients victimized by the limitations of their insurance coverage. The questions concerning how far a hospital or health system must extend its fiscal resources to promote health care equity for patients whose resources and access to health are limited by unjust circumstances are perennial, and are even more strongly represented in this edition. The first edition was among the first publications in bioethics to identify the theme of "discharge dilemmas," which are caused at least in part by the emerging (and continuing) emphasis on reducing the length of stay in a hospital. This theme is again prominent in the organizational ethics section and, to a great extent, in the entire book.

In sum, this new edition again addresses the everyday clinical ethics challenges that frontline clinicians face within the context of today's consolidated and reconfigured hospitals and health systems. These issues confront clinicians from many health care professions, and this book can be helpful to all of them, whether in a basic clinical ethics course or as a member of a health system's ethics committee. However, this edition has been especially configured and developed in conjunction with online content aimed at persons who seek to enhance their skills as clinical ethics consultants.

Developing Clinical Ethics Case Consultation Skills

A clinical ethics consultant needs well-developed knowledge, skills, and appropriate attitudes. The features of this book can assist a potential consultant with each of these facets of their professional development.

We provide a brief "conceptual framework," with several references for further reading, at the end of each of the book's four sections. Although such brief discourses on informed consent and capacity, end-of-life decision making, decision making for minors, and organizational ethics cannot replace the more extensive training available through graduate coursework, they provide sufficient context to understand the ethical foundations that typically underpin mainstream thinking concerning clinical ethics cases such as the challenging ones provided. We help the reader bring this framework closer to application in each case by also providing a "practical commentary and cheat sheet" at the end of each section. These subsections also provide tips to keep in mind when approaching such specific cases. They include possible strategies and sometimes highlight particular biases or attitudes that might be undermining progress in the case. These subsections do not provide any "answers" to the problems in the cases. Instead, they provide suggestions for significant preparation before initiating the clinical ethics consultation process.

This casebook, and the correlative online materials available on the website of Loyola University Chicago's Neiswanger Institute for Bioethics and Health Policy, also make it possible to improve one's interpersonal skills in conducting a clinical ethics case consultation. Many who wish to conduct such a consultation find it difficult to secure sufficient training opportunities to develop these skills in practice. To address this deficit, we provide the materials for simulated ethics consultations that facilitate and promote the development of the interpersonal skills that are crucial for effectively conducting ethics consultations. Each section begins with a skill builder case that is formatted to be used in role play exercises or full-scale simulations. Each character in the simulation receives a series of motivations on which to base their performance. The ethics consultant receives points to keep in mind, and may supplement their knowledge base from the extended ethical analysis that is provided for each skill builder case.

We urge users of this text to access the correlative videos and assessment tool available on the Assessing Clinical Ethics Skills (ACES) pages of Loyola University Chicago's Neiswanger Institute for Bioethics and Health Policy. The ACES project (http://LUC .edu/ethicsconsult/) provides video simulations of the skill builder cases and an assessment tool that you can use to evaluate the performance of the clinical ethics consultant in each video. A scoring rubric is provided on the website to inform users on how to apply the ACES tool to each case. After scoring the videos, you can see how your evaluation compares with those of an expert panel of ethics consultants, and you can also receive an explanation of why the panelists scored the video the way they did. As you grow in familiarity with the assessment tool, you will come to see that it is a guide to the skills that the clinical ethics consultant must accomplish or demonstrate as part of a competently conducted clinical ethics consultation. Thus, scoring the videos is also good preparation for doing your own simulations in which you practice your interpersonal clinical ethics consultation skills.

Using the ACES website requires only that you register by completing the demographic data sought when you click on the "Request Access" link. The materials are then made available free of charge. By registering with the site, you contribute to the further development and refinement of these materials. Your responses will help the "experts" learn how others see the performance.

We believe that a wide variety of users will find the second edition of this book and the online materials amenable to their specific needs. In particular, each user or group of users can develop their knowledge, skills, and attitudes in a manner and at a pace that are comfortable for them. Those who are just beginning on the path of clinical ethics, such as new hospital ethics committee members, can use the written cases and the practical commentaries and theoretical frameworks to build their knowledge foundations. Those who are beginning to conduct clinical ethics case consultations can use the skill builder cases and the correlative online ACES tool to deepen their understanding of the goals of a clinical ethics consultation. Ultimately, participating directly in simulated cases and assessing performance are likely to be important ways to improve one's skills, competence, and confidence.

Welcome to the Living Casebook

Any book of this type is by its nature incomplete. Many additional kinds of cases, with their nuanced ethical issues, could have been included. And each year, new kinds of cases arise. Rather than attempt to make this edition exhaustive, we will continue adding to the casebook in virtual fashion.

As we have mentioned, the website of the ACES project of the Neiswanger Institute for Bioethics and Health Policy at Loyola University Chicago contains video simulations of the skill builder cases that begin each section of this book. Over time, additional video simulations and materials to enact the simulated ethics cases that are not part of this book will be added. In addition, several times a year, we will post new, interesting cases with commentaries by experts and host webinars to discuss such cases. This material will be available free of charge to users who register with the site. We hope to continue to build on the foundation that was first laid in these pages in 1999 and that has been refined in this edition.

The concept of this book's life and development also embodies a significant amount of humility. We have never presumed that only certain kinds of cases or issues are ethically interesting or relevant. We did not set out to get certain kinds of cases for this book. That people reported these cases to us as ethically challenging means that they are by definition interesting and relevant. Although we have embraced a certain model of ethics consultation in the skill builder cases and online materials, the book can also be used by persons with a different understanding of how ethics works in the hospital setting. To this end, we did not alter the original thirteen cases from the first edition to fit our model. You will notice that many of these cases do not involve an ethics consultant at all. Also, we retain the original language that was used by some to reflect their process—for example, an "ethics review team." We believe that there remains a range of ways to conceive of clinical ethics activity and that we should not superimpose the current dominant understanding as if it were the only approach. As additional models of clinical ethics services surface or evolve, we hope to feature them in new materials on the ACES website, http://LUC.edu/ethicsconsult/.

References

American Society for Bioethics and Humanities. 2011. *Core Competencies for Healthcare Ethics Consultation*, 2nd edition. Chicago: American Society for Bioethics and Humanities.

Fins, J. J., E. Kodish, C. Braddock, F. Cohn, N. N. Dubler, A. Derse, R. A. Pearlman, M. Smith, A. Tarzian, S. Youngner, and M. G. Kuczewski. 2013. "Quality Attestation for Clinical Ethics Consultants: A Two-Step Model from the American Society for Bioethics and Humanities." *Hastings Center Report* 43, no. 5: 26–36.

Fins, J. J., E. Kodish, F. Cohn, M. Danis, A. R. Derse, N. N. Dubler, B. Goulden, M. Kuczewski, M. B. Mercer, R. A. Pearlman, M. L. Smith, A. Tarzian, and S. J. Youngner. 2016."A Pilot Evaluation of Portfolios for Quality Attestation of Clinical Ethics Consultants." *American Journal of Bioethics* 16, no. 3: 15–24.

Acknowledgments

We wish to thank all who have made the correlative online resources of the ACES project possible. We wish to thank our Loyola University Chicago Stritch School of Medicine colleagues—Michael McCarthy, PhD, and Kayhan Parsi, JD, PhD—for the many hours spent working with us to develop and refine the content of the ACES scoring tool. Viva Jo Siddal, MS, MS, RRT, RCP, and William Adams, MA, provided the technical expertise that guided the construction and refinement of the tool. The impressive website of the ACES project owes almost entirely to the innovative work and persistence of Bob Johnson, MEd, and Rejoice Jebamalaidass, MBA.

We again recall the contributions of several sources to the first edition of the casebook. The generous support of the Vira I. Heinz Endowment was integral to its inception. We also recall the assistance Ms. Jody Chidester Stockdill and Mr. Ryan Sauder gave in the preparation of the original manuscript. The exercise that gave rise to the book, a participant-driven educational exercise in continuing medical ethics, was initially suggested in 1992 by the Consortium Ethics Program's former consortium ethicist, Gretchen Aumann, RN, MSN, and by Anne Medsgar, RN, MS, an evaluation consultant. We thank them for having suggested the concept.

One of the cases included in the first edition and reprinted here formed the basis of a journal article. We wish to thank the relevant editors and publishers for permission to reprint the case: Mark G. Kuczewski, "Reconceiving the Family: The Process of Consent in Medical Decision Making," *Hastings Center Report* 26, no. 2 (1996): 30–37.

Acknowledgments

Our deepest debt of gratitude belongs to all those who contributed cases. Obviously, without their generosity, this book would not have been possible. In alphabetical order follow the names of those who identified cases for this book. We wish to express our thanks to each for sharing his or her experience: Judith S. Black, MD; Andrew Bonwit, MD; Patricia Cassidy, MBA; Elizabeth Chaitin, MSW, MA; Darlette Cimino, RN; Ann Lau Clark, MSN; Michael DeVita, MD; Patty Eppinger, CMSC; Maryanne Fello, RN, BSN, MEd; Jeffrey Frye, MD; Marianne Garrity, RN; Karen Gelston, MSW; Jeanne Graff, MSN; Patricia Hillebrand, RN, CNS; Sandra Janaszek, RN, MSN; Mary Johnson, RN; Elayne Krahe, BSPA; Fran Kuhns, MSN; Leah Laffey, RN, MSN; Mary Jane Lesnick-Mertz, LSW, ACSW; John Lipson, MD, MBA; Carol Lukoff, MSW; Susan McCarthy, MA; Patrick J. McCruden, MTS, D. Bioethics; Elizabeth Moore, MSW; Cynthiane J. Morgenweck, MD, MA; Alice Moskowitz; Teresa Nolan, MD; Joan Nypaver, BSN, CRRN; Margaret Pavelek, RN, BSN; William Prenatt, MD; Deborah Price, RN, BSN, MHA; Valerie Satkoske, MSW, PhD; Sarah Schlieper, LSW, CCM; Jacqueline Sikina, RN; Tom Sobieralski, MA; Sandy Thorpe, RN; Andrew Thurman, JD, MPH (deceased); Lillian Vendig-Bandyk, MSW, MPH; Philip Williams, MDiv, STM; and Mary Ellen Wyszomierski, MD.

SECTION I

CONSENT AND CAPACITY

Case 1:
Truth Telling and Culture—
Using an Interpreter in a Consultation

SKILL BUILDER CASE: This case is designed for building clinical ethics consultation skills through simulation. Visit the ACES website for a video enacting this consultation and skills assessment materials at LUC.edu/ethicsconsult/.

Key Terms: *Patient Autonomy, Decision-Making Capacity, Competence, Cultural Competence, Culturally Appropriate Care, Cultural Awareness, Cultural Sensitivity, Informed Consent, Interpreter Services, Surrogate Decision Making, Family Integrity, Truth Telling, Waiver of Informed Consent*

Narrative

The patient, Lucia Ramirez, is a sixty-five-year-old woman of Mexican descent. She has lived in the United States for about fifteen years, having moved to join her children. She speaks some words of English but is of limited English proficiency. Her oldest daughter, Ines, accompanies her to all her medical visits and serves as her translator. Mr. Ramirez died about three years ago, after a long course of emphysema and congestive heart failure.

Mrs. Ramirez presented with a large growth in the soft tissue in her lower torso. She was initially told through her daughter that the growth would need to be biopsied. Depending on what the lab analysis showed from the biopsy, the diagnosis would be made and decisions concerning courses of treatment—such as surgery, chemotherapy, and radiation—would be made. No prognosis could be offered until that diagnosis was made.

Ines informed the attending physician and the nurse manager that they must not give further bad news to Mrs. Ramirez if there was any to give. That is, all bad news should be given to Ines, who would then give encouraging news to her mother. She explained that in her culture it was common to protect one's parents, especially their mother, from bad news that would potentially devastate her (Ines said news of serious cancer would "kill" her). Ines believes she could get her mother to all needed treatments by explaining that she would be "cured" of whatever she had by the treatments. The attending physician explained that he needed to call the hospital's ethics committee, which would send someone over to talk with them.

Perspectives for Role Players

Dr. Hutchison [played by a physician or actor]:

- You are an internist who has seen Mrs. Ramirez a couple of times in the past, but you have not really established much of a connection yet.
- You are board-certified in your specialty of geriatrics and are soon likely to be consulting an oncologist once the biopsy is done. It is likely that the oncologist will take over her care for a while.

- You would like to get this decision-making process sorted out before getting the oncologist involved.
- You consider it unprofessional to "turf" this problem to the oncologist without addressing it.
- You generally believe in telling patients the truth, but you often say that you do not like to "beat patients over the head" with bad news.
- Therefore, you are open to any sort of compromise that can be worked out, as long as it is within established norms for this sort of thing. You are unsure about the ethics of this kind of scenario or your legal obligations. As a result, you would like ethics to make a recommendation, and you would likely follow it.

Ines Gomez (the patient's daughter) [played by an actor]:

- You simply want to help your mother. You feel she gets very emotional when she hears bad things, and it is your job to take care of her.
- Your father always told you that your mother was not strong and you would need to take care of her when he was gone.
- You do not really understand why the doctor would hesitate in responding to your request. After all, he wants what is best for the patient, right?
- And you certainly have some friends whose doctors have agreed to such requests.
- When your father was sick, your mother occasionally said that "in the old country, they didn't tell the patient so much. Maybe it was better."
- You do not want to make the doctor angry, and you will probably agree with what he says in the end. He is the doctor. But you want to be sure he really hears what you are saying

before you agree. Those doctors often do not listen very much to what families say.

- You are open to getting insulted by this ethics person—you are not sure what they do or why they are here. But you have an idea they do not trust you, and you do not trust them.

Ethics Consultant [played by you]:

- You have a simple principle you wish to see honored. Patients must either be told the truth or they must explicitly waive their right to information.
- You want the physician to understand that he cannot simply agree to withhold the truth from this patient.
- You are open to having someone ask Mrs. Ramirez if she would like her test results given to her daughter and having Ines make decisions so that Mrs. Ramirez can just focus on caring for herself (i.e., waiver by the patient of informed consent).
- You are concerned that because Ines is the interpreter, she might simply withhold the truth anyway.
- Therefore, you are interested in having one of your Spanish-speaking interpreters be present when the test results are given, to help with the "technical aspects" of translation, or having one of them follow up on the case afterward.

Ethical Analysis

This case presents the dilemma of informing the patient of her (cancer) diagnosis directly versus not disclosing the results of the biopsy directly—namely, omitting the word "cancer" from discussions. Ines Gomez believes that breaking any bad news to her mother would do harm. Ines is adamant that in Mexican culture, patients are protected from bad news to allow them to focus on "getting better" and remaining hopeful. Telling Mrs. Ramirez that she has cancer would deflate any hope she has and, in essence (psychologically), take away any reason she has to fight the disease and live. Ines wants the ethics consultant to understand her cultural values and recognize their importance for both her and her mother. The physician is concerned that he is being asked to be less than truthful with his patient or to lie to her, albeit a lie of omission, which makes him very uneasy. Once the biopsy is returned, if it is not cancer, then he will tell Mrs. Ramirez the good news. If it is a cancer diagnosis, he does not believe it is right to withhold this information from his patient. In fact, he knows he has a duty to inform Mrs. Ramirez of her condition and ask about her wishes for treatment.

Ethically, two different but related duties are relevant to this case. The first is the duty of disclosure. A physician is obligated to disclose the patient's diagnosis that precedes discussion of treatment options and recommendations. Without the disclosure of the patient's condition, fully informed, valid consent is not possible. This standard of informed consent means that a patient with decision-making capacity must be informed of his or her diagnosis, prognosis, and treatment options in order to make an informed choice. According to the doctrine of informed consent, a physician or other health care professional cannot touch a patient without the patient's consent, or else the physician commits battery. Such consent may be implicit, as the patient holds her arm out for a blood draw, or explicit, as she verbally agrees to have her blood pressure measured or to undergo surgery.

The second duty of the physician to his or her patient is that of truth telling. If the physician withholds information about Mrs. Ramirez's diagnosis—for example, that it is cancer—then he is violating the trust placed in him and the duty to be truthful with her. To be less than truthful means the patient may make decisions based on inaccurate or incomplete information that may lead to significant harm. In Western cultures, the patient is to be given information about his or her medical condition directly and accurately. Withholding a cancer diagnosis would not be ethically appropriate or justifiable.

One reason that fully informed, valid consent is valued in health care is that it respects the autonomy of the patient. What Mrs. Ramirez would want in the face of a cancer diagnosis is crucial to determining how the team will move forward. She will have multiple options for treatment and may need time to process the information; but ultimately, she will be able to choose the next steps in her care. The doctrine of informed consent also includes the ability to refuse medical interventions. In order to consent to a treatment, or refuse it, a patient must understand the risks, benefits, and alternatives of that treatment. In order for the treatments to be explained, the patient needs to be told about his or her underlying condition. A patient with decision-making capacity may refuse any or all treatment options, but not without a clear understanding of his or her medical condition.

The challenge for the ethics consultant in this case is that Ines Gomez, and apparently her mother, come from a very different culture, where patients are often not informed of their medical conditions, particularly if it is bad news. Patients are shielded from any negative news and may be unaware of their underlying diagnosis. Omitting a "bad" diagnosis is seen as protecting the patient from becoming discouraged and "giving up hope." The patient is then able to hold on to the belief that she will recover and concentrate her energy on getting better. Ines may argue that this approach is the compassionate one. One key role of the ethics consultant is to ensure that all parties are able to express these values, while also being clear that the options proposed are ethically justifiable and within the accepted standards set in clinical practice.

The clash of values in this case is between the duties of disclosure and truth telling on the part of the physician, and the harm that may ensue if these are not upheld, versus protecting the patient from hearing bad news. Ethically, Dr. Murphy must attempt to inform Mrs. Ramirez of her diagnosis and ask if she wishes to receive further information about her condition or not. If not, Mrs. Ramirez can indicate that she wants Ines, or someone else, to make decision for her and be the conduit of any updates and changes. Patients may choose to opt out of receiving information about their condition, and they may select a surrogate to communicate and, potentially, make decisions on their behalf even if they have capacity. This is called "waiving" one's informed consent rights. If this were the case, such discussions and the waiver decision would need to be carefully documented in the notes. Alternatively, Mrs. Ramirez may surprise her daughter and want to be actively involved in decisions about her care and treatment. Although this outcome may seem unlikely, the ethics consultant must be careful not to assume that different cultural paradigms apply to all patients and families from that culture. Communicating with the patient directly is the gold standard, and a key element of any treatment decision.

Case 2:
What Does She *Really* Want?
Coercion, Persuasion, and the Family

Key Terms: *Autonomy, Decision-Making Capacity, Competence, Informed Consent, Surrogate Decision Making, Family Autonomy*

Narrative

Mrs. L was a fifty-year-old woman who was transferred to a tertiary care facility from a primary care hospital. She had a husband who visited frequently, if not daily. She also had several brothers and sisters, but no children. Mrs. L was currently suffering from multiple external lacerations on her hands, chest, and groin area along with kidney failure. These health problems were related to her long-term, insulin-dependent diabetes. She has suffered from diabetes since childhood, but the complications and consequences of this illness have increased recently, with a leg amputation being necessary about a year ago. She began dialysis shortly thereafter.

Mrs. L was transferred to the tertiary care facility to have the lesions biopsied for diagnostic purposes. The lesions were open,

---

Versions of this case, accompanied by variations in the commentary, have been previously published in two venues: Kuczewski 1996; and Kuczewski 1997, 143–44.

draining, and very painful to the patient. Initial workups ruled out vasculitis as the causal agent. Finding the source of the lesions proved difficult, and the hospitalization became prolonged as other complications developed. Mrs. L was in great pain and was given a patient-controlled analgesia machine to help provide relief. Despite these measures, pain continued to be a factor in the slow process of diagnostic testing.

After ten days of hospitalization—which included a variety of diagnostic tests and the treatment of many complications, including adjustment disorders and depressive moods—Mrs. L required surgery for perforation of gastric ulcers. She was placed in the intensive care unit (ICU) postoperatively because of atrial fibrillation, and she remained intubated. After six days in the ICU, she was extubated. The patient, however, refused to be suctioned by the nursing staff after extubation. She was transferred out of the ICU ten days after her admission to that unit.

Mrs. L began to ask the nurses to stop dialysis. These requests began about a week into this hospitalization and continued at intervals. Each time a request was made, a discussion would be held with Mrs. L, her husband, and the attending physician. In these meetings, Mr. L would often ask Mrs. L to change her mind "for him" regarding the dialysis or other tests she was resisting. Each time, the request was granted by the patient after some resistance. On a couple of occasions, the patient agreed to further diagnostic work if her husband could be with her during the test. The nursing staff became increasingly unnerved by the situation because Mrs. L would often continue to tell the nurses that she "really" wished to stop and "just wanted to die in peace." This particular wish was always superseded by the results of the patient–husband–physician conferences.

The patient and her husband grew tired of the long hospital stay. However, neither discharge to their home nor transfer back to the primary care facility near their home was ever seriously considered as a treatment option. At one conference, it was explained to the patient that transfer to another facility might entail some of the painful diagnostic tests being repeated. This information ended all further requests for a transfer.

The Language and Issues of the Case

The stability of the patient's treatment wishes is clearly at issue. Because she wavers in her statements regarding her wishes, we are not sure whether to question her decision-making capacity or to focus on possible coercion by Mr. L. The patient's autonomy is at issue, in that we are not sure if there is a question of her ability to consent, although that seems unlikely. The issue seems to be more of a concern for what respecting her autonomy will mean in this case. Several questions are clearly on the mind of the nursing staff:

1. Which of Mrs. L's wishes are her "real" ones—for example, what she tells the nurses or those to which she agrees in conference with her husband and physician?
2. Is the patient being coerced by the pressures implicit in the conference discussions, or are the wishes she expresses to the nurses off-the-cuff comments that should not be taken seriously?
3. Do family members (e.g., Mr. L) have a legitimate right to have their views made a part of the treatment decisions?
4. Does the lack of diagnostic certainty mean that we should err in the direction of preserving life? Or, does the great suffering this patient has endured make her desire to stop treatment more important than the desire to diagnose and help the patient? That is, what is in the patient's best interest?
5. Should the lack of diagnostic certainty lead us to set a high threshold of patient decision-making capacity before agreeing to terminate life-sustaining treatment?

Case 2: What Does She *Really* Want?

Perspectives and Key Points of View

Mrs. L: Her views of treatment seem to vacillate somewhat, depending on the degree of pain she feels, the level of optimism regarding restoration of health (i.e., relief from the lesions), and the parties she is addressing (husband or nursing staff). There is more we would like to know about her. For instance, when she asks her husband to be with her during diagnostic testing, is this because his presence makes the test bearable or because she hopes he will be persuaded by witnessing her suffering? Nevertheless, it is becoming clear that she does not find a life in the hospital, suffering greatly from the open lesions, to be valuable or acceptable.

Mr. L: He clearly loves his wife, and his deep attachment to her is manifest by the amount of time he spends at her side in the hospital, including helping her through difficult and painful diagnostic tests. There is a question being raised by the nursing staff as to whether he truly has her best interest at heart or is merely serving his own interests and fear of abandonment.

The attending physician: The physician initially hoped to make a quick diagnosis of the lesions and provide treatment to relieve this source of pain. As such, he had little trouble during the early part of the hospital course imparting hope to the patient and her husband and counseling that withdrawal of treatment be postponed in favor of diagnostic progress. Because the diagnosis proved to be elusive, the physician began to worry that he had misled the patient and her husband. Nevertheless, he feared that the patient's wishes to stop dialysis could be temporary expressions of pain that would pass when she was enjoying time with her husband.

It was also an initial hypothesis of the attending physician that some of Mrs. L's statements regarding the desire to stop treatment emanated from fear of abandonment and that she made these statements to elicit commitment from her husband. However, this hypothesis dissipated with time, and the physician became increasingly concerned about how to reconcile the feelings of the patient and those of her husband.

The nursing staff: The nurses are convinced that they know that the patient "really" wishes to stop dialysis and die peacefully. The nurses believe that the physician should take the patient's statements to them as definitive of her wishes and not subject her to the "coercion" of the three-way conferences.

What Actually Happened

Several weeks into her hospitalization, Mrs. L remained adamant in her treatment refusals during the conference with her husband and physician. Mr. L then agreed to accept her wishes and agreed to stay by her during her death. The physician wrote a do-not-resuscitate order and an order to discontinue dialysis. Palliative care continued to be provided. The patient died within forty-eight hours, accompanied by her grieving husband.

Case 3:
"He Doesn't Know What He's Saying"
Advance Directives
in Emergency Settings

Key Terms: *Autonomy, Decision-Making Capacity, Competence, Informed Consent, Surrogate Decision Making, Advance Directives, Emergency Department Ethics, Physician Order for Life-Sustaining Treatment (POLST)*

Narrative

Mr. J, a sixty-five-year-old married man, presented at the emergency room in acute respiratory distress. He was anxious, alert, and gasping for air. His shortness of breath made talking with him difficult. He was accompanied by his wife and nephew.

Mr. J was fairly well known at this hospital because he had been treated there for almost a decade for his chronic pulmonary disease. His illness progressed over the years to the point where he required assistance dressing and eating, and this assistance was provided by his wife, who cared for him at home. Mr. J had been admitted to the hospital ten months before, at which time he was intubated and placed on a respirator. Later, there was great difficulty weaning the patient from the machine, but the pulmonologist managed to do so after two weeks. According to the family, Mr. J expressed strong feelings at that time that he should never be placed on a ventilator again.

During the current presentation, Mrs. J and her nephew spoke with the attending physician in the Emergency Department while Mr. J was taken to the treatment room. They explained what they believed to be the patient's wishes. That is, they asked that Mr. J be given any helpful medications but not be intubated. They also asked that his code status be "do not resuscitate." The family said that Mr. J should be made "comfortable" and that necessary medications could be given to him.

The family did not enter the treatment room with the physician. The physician examined the patient; and in the presence of the nursing staff and respiratory therapists, the physician explained the need for intubation to Mr. J, who agreed to this by nodding his head "yes." This process took place quickly due to the emergency conditions. Mr. J was intubated and placed on a ventilator within ten minutes of admission. Upon learning of the intubation, the family became very upset.

The Language and Issues of the Case

Several problems are evident. Clearly, this case will be discussed in terms of the patient's right to make his own decision—that is, patient autonomy. But whether this is an autonomous decision will require placing several matters in context:

1. Determining the patient's capacity to consent to treatment ("decision-making capacity" or "competence");
2. Identifying the role of previous directions ("advance directives") in treatment decisions; and

3. Deciding the role of family or surrogates in interpreting the wishes of a patient.

Perspectives and Key Points of View

Emergency room physician: The physician was reluctant to take the family's initial request at face value. He believed that a patient who presents at the emergency room should receive the kind of care that is standard in such emergency situations. Thus, he has the normal presumption to treat in the emergency situation. Furthermore, he was also reluctant to give the family's request priority because the patient was conscious. Although the patient's decision-making capacity is at issue, the physician believed that he should presume the patient to be competent to consent to life-saving interventions unless clearly shown otherwise. After the fact, the physician wondered whether he had done the right thing.

The family (Mrs. J and nephew): The family members believed that they knew the patient's real wishes because they had a long period during which to discuss the future course of treatment. They also believed that if Mr. J contradicted what they believed to be his genuine wishes, it must be due to hypoxia or the coercive atmosphere of the treatment room. They dreaded the possibility that the prolonged agony of the previous difficult weaning period would be repeated. Mr. J was generally conscious during those attempts, and they watched the patient linger in fear and suffering for two weeks. They also feared that they would be "killing" Mr. J if they withdrew the respirator after unsuccessful weaning attempts. In contrast, they also believed that it would have been acceptable if Mr. J had not been started on the mechanical ventilator in the first place. They felt that the emergency room physician had betrayed them and undermined their familial role as the interpreters of the patient's wishes.

What Actually Happened

No information is available on the outcome of this case. See the notes in our cheat sheet and tips at the end of the chapter for more thoughts on how a clinical ethics consultant might approach it.

Case 4:
"Please Don't Cut Off My Leg"
Going from a Wish to a Plan of Care

Key Terms: *Autonomy, Surrogate Decision Making*

Narrative

Mr. R was a fifty-seven-year-old man with diabetes mellitus, hypertension, and severe peripheral vascular disease. Mr. R was morbidly obese, and his left leg manifested arteriole insufficiency for several years. The patient has now been admitted for a gangrenous left foot. He previously had surgery for revascularization, but this clearly had not been able to solve the long-term problem. The patient also has ulcers on his right foot. A course of intravenous (IV) antibiotics was begun to treat the infection.

The attending physician sought a surgical consultation, and both physicians agreed that an amputation of the left leg below the knee was indicated. Both believed that the gangrene would eventually take the patient's life unless the limb was amputated. They explained this to the patient, who simply refused. However, the patient's responses to the physicians' questions were not directly responsive and were somewhat irrational. For instance, he kept simply asserting that he did not want his leg cut off and that the physicians and everyone at the hospital were "racist." Two of the patient's adult brothers where present for this conversation and tried to interject to the patient that the doctors were "just trying to help him" and that he should "listen to them." Nevertheless, no plan of care was able to be explored in any detail during this initial conversation. The surgeon and the attending physician said that they would come back the following day for a follow-up conversation. The attending physician paged the ethics consultant and asked that he also sit in on the meeting the next morning.

During the next day's conversation, the patient was more engaging of the prognosis. He clearly was fearful of having part of his leg removed; and at one point, in a low voice, he said, "Please don't cut off my leg." The attending physician explained that this was needed if the patient was to live for an extended period. Nevertheless, he also pointed out that the patient had a fair number of comorbidities and that the patient's other foot could progress in the same way in the future. As a result, the ethics consultant who was present for this conversation suggested that the choice at this point might be better to focus on goals of care—for example, life extension versus palliation—rather than on particular interventions.

The Language and Issues of the Case

This case in some ways is the most straightforward kind of informed consent case. The patient gets to be informed of his options and make a decision. From the description of the patient, his decision-making capacity does not seem to be impaired. Nevertheless,

1. What will it mean for this patient to be adequately informed? That is, how can he come to appreciate what life postamputation would be like? And how could he come to appreciate what death from the gangrenous foot would be like with support from a hospice service?

2. What role does fear of the unknown—that is, life without one's leg—play in this kind of decision? How can such fears be placed in proper perspective?

Perspectives and Key Points of View

Mr. R: The patient had struggled with his health difficulties for a very long time. Although he was not depressed and wished to go on living, because there were a number of things that he enjoyed doing in daily life, he was terrified of starting to lose limbs to amputation. In particular, he was worried that the limited mobility that would follow would make him increasingly dependent on his family, especially if he ended up having both feet eventually amputated.

The attending physician: The attending physician had seen many patients who had a below-knee amputation done owing to peripheral vascular disease. In general, he very much favored such a procedure, as it often resulted in a good quality of life for an extended period for his patients. However, in this case, he was more ambivalent because the patient's medical problems would likely result in a continued diminishment of his quality of life. Thus, the physician hoped that the patient might begin to wrestle with the big picture of what he would want.

The surgeon: The surgeon was surprised that there was much debate about what to do. He believed strongly in doing a below-knee amputation in this situation because it seemed to him that death from the progression of gangrene was a very undesirable way to die.

The ethics consultant: The ethics consultant was initially concerned about the role that fear might be playing in the patient's decision making process. When he was told of the initial conversation with the patient, it seemed that the patient might "shut down" rather than engage the issues. The consultant hoped that they might be able to consider the long-term picture of what the patient's life might be like after an amputation and what the patient might expect to happen thereafter.

What Actually Happened

The discussion between the patient, the physicians, and the ethics consultant resulted in the patient tentatively deciding that he would like to pursue palliation rather than surgery. However, he wished to speak with a palliative care consultant and the hospice intake director. Mr. R wanted to get a clearer picture of how his discomfort would be managed and what his dying process would be like. He met with these persons the following day and was discharged to his home with hospice care within forty-eight hours.

Case 5:
Consent and the Elderly—
Is the Patient Her Own
Best Spokesperson?

Key Terms: *Ageism, Competence, Decision-Making Capacity, Informed Consent, Competence, Power of Attorney, Durable Power of Attorney for Health Care (DPAHC)*

Narrative

Mrs. F is an eighty-four-year-old resident of a local nursing facility who was evaluated in the emergency room after sustaining a fall in the bathroom. She has had multiple medical problems in the past, none of which have been particularly debilitating. She has a history of hypertension, depression, arthritis, and hyperthyroidism, and she has been given a vague diagnosis of senile dementia.

Upon falling in the bathroom, Mrs. F apparently struck her head and sustained a large hematoma and a laceration. She was evaluated by the staff of the nursing facility and was found to be alert and oriented. Because of the laceration, she was transferred to the emergency room for evaluation. In the emergency room, a routine computed tomography scan of her head was obtained and revealed a rather large subdural hematoma compressing the ventricles and pushing on the brain. In spite of this finding, Mrs. F seemed to be her usual self and was aware that she was in the emergency room

— 23 —

and was conversing easily with the staff there. It was explained to her that she had a condition that could not be treated at the community hospital and that she required transfer to a tertiary care facility. She accepted this and told the emergency room physician that it would be OK to transfer her.

On arrival at the emergency room of the tertiary care facility, Mrs. F was evaluated by a neurosurgeon. At that time, the patient was complaining of a headache. She related that she knew she was at a different hospital and was not in the nursing home. She was unable to give any details as to what had happened to her, but she was able to relay that she had fallen and struck her head. Neurological examination revealed that she had decreased motor strength of the right side and somewhat garbled speech. The neurosurgeon needed to determine whether Mrs. F should undergo a burr hole to drain her subdural hematoma to relieve the pressure on the brain or return her to the nursing home and monitor her in the hope that the clot would resolve.

While staying at the nursing home, Mrs. F was noted by the staff to be an alert and gregarious elderly woman who "got around" well. She performed most of her activities of daily living with minimal assistance. She was oriented at all times. While at the nursing home, she had completed an advance directive, which stated that "if she were ever terminally ill or permanently unconscious, life-prolonging measures such as cardiac resuscitation, ventilatory support, and artificial nutrition and hydration should be withheld." The patient also requested comfort measures if she should become debilitated. Mrs. F designated her nephew as her power of attorney. The power of attorney was solely for financial transactions and did not impart health care decision-making powers to the nephew. Discovered after the fact was that Mrs. F had a sister. Unfortunately, the staff at the nursing home facility were unaware of this sister's existence. Mrs. F's husband was deceased, and she had no children.

Case 5: Consent and the Elderly

At this point, the neurosurgeon elected to contact the family member who held Mrs. F's power of attorney: her nephew, whom the neurosurgeon believed was her only living relative. The neurosurgeon discussed Mrs. F's case with her nephew at some length, and relayed to him that Mrs. F had an advance directive. He explained the critical nature of Mrs. F's condition and the potentially devastating outcome if surgery were not performed.

Mrs. F's nephew was unsure how to proceed at that time. It was not clear that he understood the gravity of the situation or the fact that a burr hole would relieve the pressure on Mrs. F's brain. At this point, a decision was made to return the patient to the nursing home on anticonvulsant medications and to perform no surgical intervention.

The Language and Issues of the Care

This case raises a variety of issues, depending on the point in Mrs. F's treatment on which one focuses and on whom one focuses—for example, the neurosurgeon, the patient's attending physician, and the nursing home staff. Questions of informed consent loom large early, and then questions regarding decision-making capacity and the naming of an appropriate surrogate take precedence later. Thus, one can ask:

1. Is a surrogate decision maker necessary in this case, or was Mrs. F's autonomy violated by not being included in a discussion of her medical condition and potential treatments?
2. If a surrogate decision maker was necessary, was the appropriate surrogate Mrs. F's nephew, who was her power of attorney for financial matters?
3. Did the neurosurgeon in this case make a prejudiced determination of Mrs. F's quality of life before her fall, and thereby

base decisions on faulty assumptions about her? Or was he practicing the standard of care for the treatment of a hematoma in a patient of her age?

4. Were there others in this patient's life—for example, the nursing home staff and her primary care physician—who should have played a larger role in the decision-making process?

Perspectives and Key Points of View

The patient: We have no idea what she actually thought. She was not really asked.

The nursing home staff: The staff who knew Mrs. F at the nursing home described her as capable of making her own decisions because she was always quite conversant and self-directing. They were outraged that the patient did not undergo surgery and that they were left out of the decision-making process. They also now have an added burden: to monitor her closely while the clot is resolving.

The nephew: He was the financial power of attorney and was not comfortable with being asked to make health care decisions concerning his aunt. It was his feeling that the health care decisions should be left up to the physicians involved and that they would know best what to do for his aunt.

The neurosurgeon: He believed the patient was incompetent to make treatment decisions, and he felt burdened because he had to lead the patient's surrogate in making a decision to operate or not. The nephew did not have a clear preference, so the neurosurgeon believed he must provide the decision. He did not think she was a good candidate for surgery and he also knew that, given time, the clot could resolve without further harm to the patient.

What Actually Happened

Mrs. F was returned to the nursing home facility. One day later, she was evaluated by her primary care physician. At that time, she was semicomatose. She was totally paralyzed on her right side and had a ragged breathing pattern. To discuss her condition, the attending physician contacted Mrs. F's nephew, who said that he wanted her to undergo surgery if the attending physician felt that any of the symptoms were reversible. Given her grave respiratory and neurological status, the attending physician felt that it would be inappropriate to pursue surgery. Mrs. F was therefore maintained on anticonvulsant medications and observed. In two weeks' time, Mrs. F was again able to swallow and was opening her eyes and responding to simple commands. Because there was some improvement in her condition and in subsequent computed tomography scans, a second neurosurgical consultation was obtained. This consultant's opinion was that Mrs. F's subdural hematoma was resolving and she would not require surgery. After one month, Mrs. F was able to sit unassisted, was again using her right side, and was able to walk a few steps. Although not quite the same, she became alert and was oriented to her surroundings, and she was able to carry on conversations with the nursing facility staff.

Case 6:
"I Don't Want Any Tubes"
Capacity and the Care of a Patient
with a Kidney Transplant

Key Terms: *Decision-Making Capacity, Forgoing Treatment, Surrogate Decision Making, Restraints, Commodity Scarcity*

Narrative

The patient, Mrs. Z, is a sixty-year-old woman who received a kidney transplant approximately one year earlier. Her current hospitalization is for a urinary tract infection and dehydration. She had a similar hospitalization three months ago. She is characterized in the medical record as "noncompliant" with her medicines, and she does not drink enough fluids to maintain her hydration. In order to treat her infection and to rehydrate her, the hospital staff would like to place a peripherally inserted central catheter (PICC) line and also additional IV lines. These would need to remain in place for several days. The patient refuses the placement.

The ethics consultant interviewed Mrs. Z and found her very difficult to engage in any sustained conversation. Mrs. Z would only offer that she "didn't want any tubes" and that the reason was because "they hurt." She repeated this line over and over when questioned. When asked whether she understood that these interventions might help her get better and that a lack of treatment could lead to her getting worse, she would say "I don't want to talk about that." She would repeat these sentences or something similar in response to virtually any question.

She has a husband, whom she married about five years ago and who is currently in a rehabilitation facility after suffering a stroke. He has difficulty speaking, but when contacted by telephone, he said that he thought "everything should be done." Hospital staff also contacted her twenty-four-year-old son, who is going to school in another state and was her kidney donor. He says his mother's mental status has never been completely right since the transplant and deteriorates significantly when she gets an infection and is dehydrated. He says that she has been negative about treatment since the transplant but would likely have wanted this care if she were her "old self." Armed with this information, the ethics consultant asked Mrs. Z if she could say how her son felt about her decisions or why he thinks she should agree to the PICC line and IV line placements. In response, she would turn away in bed and sometimes cover her head with the sheet.

The Language and Issues of the Case

The patient's decision-making capacity is clearly at issue. She is resistant to cooperating with the ethics consultant's interview, and the consultant's discussion with the son and husband seems to confirm that she lacks the capacity to make sound medical decisions for herself. The questions concern what should happen next:

1. Who is the appropriate surrogate decision maker for this patient if she lacks capacity? Does the son's role as the organ donor compromise his ability to participate in the patient's decision-making process?
2. Can a surrogate consent to restraining the patient to treat her?

3. What should be the ethics consultant's short-term recommendations? His long-term ones?

Perspectives and Key Points of View

Mrs. Z (the patient): We have very little insight into her perspective because she seems generally unable to cooperate with explaining the rationale for her wishes, even though she seems to express preferences. However, we have "witnesses" who say that these expressions do not reflect her values as they knew them. Nevertheless, by the end of the case, we are probably able to say that this patient is tiring of the struggle to maintain her health. This is expressed by Mrs. Z after treatment and is similar to the kinds of things her son says about her.

The patient's husband: The perspective of the patient's husband was difficult to obtain in detail. He seemed to have the capacity to understand the situation when questioned by the ethics consultant, and his point of view seemed coherent and reasonable. His overall assessment of his wife's mental status since the transplant seemed consistent with that of the patient's son—that is, the dehydration and infection had rendered her unable to make her own decisions during this crisis, and her mental status since the kidney transplant had not been what it was before the transplant.

The patient's son: His perspective seemed quite mature. The ethics consultant was initially skeptical of the son's voice, given that he was the organ donor. However, the facts and analysis that this person contributed were very helpful and balanced. It was invaluable to the consultant to have the son relay that the mother's current mental status was nothing like her normal self. Also, he was able to describe how even when she is hydrated and not suffering from infections, her mental status is significantly diminished from her pretransplant state. In general, he seemed to indicate a healthy concern for being sure that all potentially effective treatments be tried, but that at some point, if his mother could not regain her desire to push on, one would likely need to honor her wishes to change the goals of treatment to comfort.

What Actually Happened

The medical situation in this case was deemed to be relatively urgent by the treating team. They felt that it was very important to address her dehydration issues quickly. The attending physician and the ethics consultant tried to interview the patient one more time, but she remained uncooperative. With the concurrence of the patient's husband and son, she was sedated and restrained and was rehydrated for several days, and her infections were treated aggressively. After five days, the restraints were removed and the sedation was lightened. The patient was not agitated, and her mental status was somewhat improved. However, she did not want to discuss long-term treatment goals. She simply said that she was tired of treatment and just wanted to get better.

The patient's son told the ethics consultant that he understood that his stepfather is legally the appropriate surrogate decision maker but that he was available to help if his stepfather found making these decisions too difficult or lost his ability to do so, owing to his own health problems.

Case 7:
Caring for a Patient Who Uses Heroin— Fairness and Professional Responsibility

---

Key Terms : *Decision-Making Capacity, Forgoing Treatment, Suicide, Health Care Ethics Committees, Health Care Ethics Consultation*

Narrative

The patient, Mr. V, is a thirty-year-old male who is admitted to the general medicine unit through the Emergency Department. He presented with severe pain on his left side and a fever. The patient has not previously been seen at this hospital. Mr. V seems to be fairly forthcoming when his history is taken. He discloses that he suffers from a substance use disorder. He says that he has recently relapsed after a period of several months, during which he refrained from using his drug of choice—heroin. Mr. V indicates that he has been hospitalized twice and has been treated for endocarditis twice before. He was initially treated with antibiotics given orally. The second time, the antibiotics were administered with an IV.

The pain on his left side was diagnosed as being due to a pleural effusion. A chest tube was placed to relieve the pressure shortly after admission. However, how to treat the infection—that is, endocarditis—that was causing the fever posed some challenges for the attending physician. The physician was currently treating the endocarditis with IV antibiotics administered through a PICC line, which provides direct venous access for an indefinite period and avoids the problems that can come with the placement of an IV line in the forearm or hand. The placement of the PICC line meant that the patient could potentially leave the hospital sooner, as he might be able to use it to administer his antimicrobial therapy himself at home. However, the patient would be on his own, and thus the line would also be available for the insertion of heroin.

Unfortunately, any intravenous line presents a temptation to someone who is addicted to IV drugs. The line presents an efficient means of administration of such drugs and can thereby provide a more intense "high" than is usually available to them. As a result, the Infectious Disease Society of America's practice guidelines counsel against the use of a PICC line for outpatient antimicrobial therapy for such patients.

A "sitter" was being provided by the hospital around the clock to watch over Mr. V and help him avoid using illegal substances. But the question of discharge was important. If all he needed was several weeks of IV antibiotics, keeping him in the hospital for that amount of time seemed unwarranted. Therefore, what were the options for discharge? Could he be sent home with the PICC line to administer his own therapy? Could he go to a long-term care facility, where he could receive his antimicrobial therapy? What about the treatment of his substance use disorder? Could the treating team insist on complying with treatment for substance abuse? How, and when, should this treatment take place?

The Language and Issues of the Case

This case presents challenges to the paradigm of shared decision making between patient and physician. The physician is usually seen as providing realistic medical options, and the patient is seen as choosing treatment based on his or her values and preferences. But substance use disorders, like other forms of mental illness, can compromise a patient's ability to safeguard his best interests and can lead him to act on short-term desires that are contrary to his ultimate values. Thus, several questions arise:

1. Should the physician offer the option of discharge to home with self-administration of antibiotics through the PICC line? Is this required by the duty to respect patient autonomy? Or does the physician's duty of beneficence require him to withhold such an option from a person with a substance use disorder such as addiction to heroin?
2. Clearly, the physician should offer support for treatment of the substance use disorder. Is the patient in any way obligated to accept this offer—for example, as a condition of treatment for his endocarditis? If the patient refuses treatment for the substance use disorder, should that change the treatment options offered for his endocarditis?

Perspectives and Key Points of View

The attending physician: The attending physician, of course, wishes to successfully treat the patient for the infection and is frustrated by the patient's behavior that undermines this goal. The physician is very concerned about potentially being culpable for the patient's death if the patient were to use the IV access he has supplied to overdose on illicit drugs. Thus, he is extremely concerned about discharge options and wishes he could find a facility that would accept the transfer of this patient. If the patient is to go home, the attending physician insists that the PICC line must first be removed.

Mr. V (the patient): The patient seems to have conflicting wishes and goals. He initially seemed rather resistant to discussion of treatment of his substance use disorder, saying that he would handle it himself. However, as his stay in the hospital progressed, he became more willing to discuss the situation and to explore options for treatment. But as with many persons who suffer from addiction issues, his belief that treatment could ever be effective waxed and waned. He was particularly interested in in-patient treatment programs because they seemed most likely to be effective to him.

Social worker (case manager): The case manager wishes to provide a safe discharge that meets the patient's medical needs, both in terms of his endocarditis and his substance use disorder. Meeting these goals is complicated by several factors, including ambivalence of the patient toward treatment for his addiction, the lack of appropriate facilities willing to take such a patient, and the willingness of the patient's insurer to reimburse facilities that might be found. She feels fortunate that the hospital's assistant chief medical officer has been briefed on the case and has made clear that the case worker should prioritize the best interest of the patient in devising a plan.

What Actually Happened

An ethics consultation resulted in several team meetings to devise a discharge plan. Based on national guidelines, the attending physician did not believe that he could discharge the patient to his home with the PICC line in place. As a result, the hospital social worker (case manager) searched for skilled nursing facilities and long-term care facilities that might accept this patient. Although few facilities felt that this patient presented a profile for which they were equipped to care, one skilled nursing facility was found that would accept the patient, and the patient's insurer agreed to cover a stay at the facility. However, before the discharge plan could be executed, the patient attempted to inject heroin into his PICC line and was discovered doing this by the sitter. As a result, the skilled nursing facility rescinded its offer of admission, leaving the hospital with no option to discharge to another facility.

The patient then agreed to treatment for his substance use disorder. The attending physician began a plan of care, with a medication known as Suboxone that is used to treat opioid addictions. The social worker began seeking in-patient treatment programs that would follow up on this care, as it was thought this patient could use the support of an in-patient environment for initial treatment. Unfortunately, no slot in any such program could be found that would be available in the foreseeable future.

The patient remained in the hospital for two months, until his antimicrobial therapy was completed and the PICC line was removed. He was discharged to his home, and he agreed to present at an outpatient substance use disorder program on the following Monday. Nothing further is known about this patient's outcome.

Practical Commentary and Tips on Informed Consent and Capacity, with a Cheat Sheet for Dealing with Cases 1 through 7

It has been said that "all of medical ethics is but a footnote to informed consent." Although this may seem an exaggeration, it conveys a fundamental insight: Contemporary biomedical ethics places the patient at the center of decision making, and in each clinical quandary, one must figure out what this positioning should mean. In complicated cases, an ethics consultant tries to facilitate a decision-making process that promotes respect for the patient's values and wishes. It is easy to say that health care professionals should do what the patient wishes. But the preceding cases make clear that determining what the patient wishes is not always a simple matter. In some way, each case represents a gloss on the question of patient wishes.

In the opening case (case 1), the patient's daughter tells the physician that she knows what the patient would want. In particular, she firmly believes that the patient would not want "bad news." In cases 2 and 3, the patients' "real" wishes are in question. Are those wishes what the patient expresses when in the company of family, or are they what the patient says to a health care provider when no one else is listening? Each of these first three cases raises the question of whether people who know the patient, such as family members, are "privileged" interpreters of patient wishes or not.

Cases 4 through 7 are scenarios in which the capacity of the patient to make decisions based on his or her wishes and to safeguard their best interest is doubtful. In such cases, patients often say something, but there seem to be good reasons to doubt that these words represent a values-based choice. In case 4, Mr. R's initial statements of refusal are not taken as seriously as his later ones because the former seem to be reactions based in fear (e.g., calling the treating team "racist"), while the latter are based on deliberation concerning his options and long-term prognosis. In cases 5 and 6, we are not sure if the patient is able to understand the long-term implications of their situation and any choices they might make. And case 7 is perhaps the most difficult of all, because addiction can impair a patient's ability to act in accord with his best interests, even if he seems to understand the situation and wishes to adhere to a plan of care.

Of course, informed consent means that the patient should be informed and educated concerning options that are consistent with the integrity of the medical profession. Cases 5 and 7 raise questions concerning what a physician should reasonably offer. The physicians would be well advised to offer and provide the standard of care. However, the standard of care is seldom a one-size-fits-all formula, but must be adjusted to fit the particular patient's circumstances. Thus a certain amount of judgment is required, and this judgment is likely to be refined through a process of conversations with other caregivers, people who know the patient well, and the patient. The fact that the patient may not ultimately possess the capacity to make the final decision does not nullify the relevance of his or her perspective.

The cheat sheet is as follows:

1. *Case 1:* In our cultural and ethical context, we cannot simply take a family member's word that a patient wants us to withhold information. It is a good idea to confront such a suggestion quickly and explain the concept of "waiver" of informed consent that will be necessary if we are to deviate from the usual plan of informed consent (Kuczewski and McCruden 2001).

2. *Case 2:* Use multiple conversations to come to a point where the patient is expressing the same wishes consistently. If the patient says different things to different people, try to bring the key parties together with the patient for a conversation. The patient's wishes need to be stable enough that they enable a treatment plan to be carried out over time. Thus, the "real" wishes of a patient will be those that survive encounters with close others and are made in conjunction with close others (Kuczewski 1996; Nelson and Nelson 1995).

3. *Case 3:* First, when in doubt, err on the side of life. You can always sort things out later and withdraw death-delaying treatment if that turns out to be the patient's wish. But as the risk to not treating is high, the patient's expressed preference is sufficient. However, even in emergency situations, one might take a moment to try to allay a patient's fears and see if that affects his or her decision. With the patient's permission, this can involve bringing family members into the treatment room (Drane 1984, 1985). Furthermore, once the patient has been stabilized, the consultant will need to try to involve the patient in decision making, unless that proves impossible due to deterioration of capacity. Communicating with patients who are ventilated and sedated can be impossible. But if there are decisions to be made,

asking the physician to lighten the sedation and making attempts to determine the patient's wishes would be important.

4. *Case 4:* Many things that are said by patients can distract from the fear of the future and the unknown that patients may experience when presented with life-altering treatment options, such as a limb amputation. Helping patients come to understand the realities of what those options are likely to entail can help the patient focus on treatment goals and make appropriate decisions (Wasson et al. 2017).

5. *Case 5:* This kind of case is simply very difficult, because it is always easy to err on the side of overtreatment; but one can just as easily fail to provide the treatment a patient might want based on assumptions incorrectly derived from advanced age. Sometimes an ethics consultant can only reiterate a goal, such as that expressed by the patient's nephew—for example, "he wanted her to undergo the surgery if the attending physician felt that any of the symptoms were reversible"—and leave it to the clinician to interpret its application (Feblowitz and Richards 2015).

6. *Case 6:* Ethicists are typically self-critical people and can find themselves ruminating as to whether the patient's verbal noncooperation with the interview is a kind of refusal of the ethics consultation or of capacity assessment that should be honored. However, when a patient's well-being is threatened by a condition such as dehydration, consultants may proceed aggressively, explaining to the patient that unless he or she can help you understand her reason for treatment refusal, you will need to recommend that someone else make this medical decision for her (Hurst 2004).

7. *Case 7:* The issue that you are trying to resolve as an ethics consultant may not be clear. On one hand, there is simply the

question of whether the physician should offer the placement of a PICC line that could enable the patient to receive his medication at home. Whether the ethics of informed consent requires this is not clear, given a professional society's recommendation against it. Thus, standard of care may simply trump your ethical analysis. The challenge for an ethics consultant is to advocate for a coherent plan of care for the patient that provides the opportunity for the patient to get all aspects of his needs addressed, including his substance use disorder (Tice et al. 2004; Mallon 2001).

Conceptual Framework

Informed consent has a long but ill-defined tradition, which has been articulated to some degree by the law courts. The tradition of informed consent begins roughly at the beginning of the twentieth century with a major legal case, *Schloendorf* (1914), which reached the US Supreme Court. This was a liability case, in which a patient was operated on without her consent. The patient, Ms. Mary Schloendorf, had consented to an examination under anesthesia but had specifically forbidden surgery. Justice Benjamin Cardozo issued a classic statement in this case: "Every human being of adult years and sound mind has a right to determine what shall be done with his own body."

The law tends to emphasize an individual's rights of liberty, self-determination, and privacy. The legal notion of informed consent seems to confer an unlimited right to patients or makes an absolute value out of the autonomy (the right to self-governance) of the individual. However, the reference that Justice Cardozo makes to "sound mind" is an implicit reference to the concept of competence or decision-making capacity. This is the concept of decision-making capacity that will smuggle a physician's duty of beneficence (the duty to do things that are good for the patient) back into the picture, to be balanced against the patient's autonomy. A patient has a right to unfettered self-determination as long as this patient is genuinely "autonomous"—that is, able to appropriately "govern" oneself. A person whose mental faculties are not up to the task of making decisions is not truly autonomous. Such persons must be protected by society. As a result, the idea of competence or decision-making capacity is a gatekeeper concept. One must pass through the gate to be in the ranks of those who can exercise their autonomy.

A determination of the patient's competence or decision-making capacity attempts to discern whether the patient merely has an unusual set of values or has lost the capacity to protect his or her own interests. If the former, we must respect the patient's wishes. If the latter, we need to proceed to find an appropriate surrogate to make the patient's health care decisions.

The Parts of Informed Consent and Decision-Making Capacity

Informed consent and decision-making capacity have generated a voluminous literature. In such a literature, one will find differing terminologies used to analyze these concepts into their component parts. But, in general, informed consent and decision-making capacity break down into certain kinds of activities and elements. The activities of informed consent fit into three kinds of categories:

- Disclosure
- Cognition
- Consent, refusal, or choice

This means that informed consent requires disclosure—that is, the giving of information regarding such things as the patient's situation, including diagnosis and prognosis, and possible interventions, including the risks or burdens and possible benefits. The patient must somehow be able to make mental use of this information, albeit according to his or her own cognitive style. Also, the patient then supplies his answer to the proposed possible interventions.

The capacity to make a choice that should be respected includes having sufficient cognitive capability to ingest the information, being able to make a choice in accordance with one's values, and being able to communicate this choice in some way so it can be understood by the clinicians.

Regarding the disclosure requirement of informed consent, there is a "how much?" question to be answered. For instance, how much information must be disclosed? In general, one can answer this by thinking about what a typical reasonable person would want to know. We can describe the risks of crossing the street in such graphic detail that it would scare anyone from ever doing it. However, most reasonable people want to know whether the cars came very fast or slowly down the street, whether there was a particularly safe place at which to cross, and why one would want to cross the street. This last question refers to the goal of crossing the street. Similarly, patients need to be clear on the goals of treatment and to formulate and revise their treatment goals in tandem with their health care provider. Patients are usually fairly good at helping to set treatment goals. Physicians are far more expert than patients at the appropriate treatments to meet these goals. Once the goals are agreed on, physicians probably do not need to be overly zealous in describing every miniscule detail of treatment. But over time, the physician comes to know which kinds of treatment the patient may find especially noxious or difficult to tolerate. She can then tailor her disclosure process to attend to these subjective concerns.

The comprehension and capacity requirements of informed consent also include "how much" issues—How competent does the patient need to be? How much must a patient comprehend? These tend to be answered relative to risk. As James Drane (1985) notes at the start of one of his articles on this topic, "The greater the risk, the higher the standard." That is, when persons are not placing themselves in harm's way with their decisions, a global presumption of their competence governs the situation. We respect their autonomy by assuming that they are autonomous beings unless they give us good reasons to doubt their capacity. Because it would be contrary to the values of our society, we will not deny a person's right to refuse treatment just because it conflicts with our values or the values of most people. But in such situations of idiosyncratic treatment refusals, one is justified in trying to be sure that the patient is capable of acting autonomously. As a result, we try to be sure that the patient definitely understands the consequences of his choice and is acting on relatively stable values.

Implementing Informed Consent: Event versus Process

There are two main models of how informed consent is done. The input–output approach we outlined above is usually thought of as an event model. Event models take place in a very discrete time period. They often involve an acute illness. The physician provides the medical facts. The patient makes a decision based on those facts. An emergency appendectomy is a good example of such a model at work. The risks of not having the surgery are clear; the benefits are also easily comprehensible.

Process models often prevail in longer-term situations—for example, chronic illness. The information that the physician provides and that the patient gathers accumulates over a period of time. Much of the information may be experiential. For instance, the patient comes to know whether he can live with a certain side effect of his medication by taking the medication and experiencing the side effect. As a result, discussions must be held more than once and issues must be revisited because the patient continually learns more about his own wishes. Information should not be one-directional. The physician comes to learn more about what the patient values, wants, and can tolerate, while the patient comes to better understand the physician's plan. Patient and physician "mutually monitor" each other. The goal is for the thinking of each to become "transparent" to the other.

In sum, one can think about the doctrine of informed consent and the theory of competence in very simple terms. That is, ideally, we want a person *to make treatment decisions the same way they generally make all important decisions in their life.* The person should think about their choices and act in a way that is consistent with their personal style, values, and the way they wish to live. If the person is unable to do this, they may need assistance to increase their capacity to do this, or the decision may need to be made by another who will act on the person's earlier wishes and values.

References and Further Reading

Drane, James F. 1984. "Competency to Give Informed Consent." *Journal of the American Medical Association* 252, no. 7: 925–27.

———. 1985. "The Many Faces of Competency." *Hastings Center Report* 15, no. 2: 17–21.

Feblowitz, Joshua, and Jeremy Richards. 2015. "What Are the Patient's Wishes?" *JAMA Internal Medicine* 175, no. 4: 490–91.

Hurst, Samia A. 2004. "When Patients Refuse Assessment of Decision-Making Capacity." *Archives of Internal Medicine* 164, no. 16: 1757–60.

Kuczewski, Mark G. 1996. "Reconceiving the Family: The Process of Consent in Medical Decision Making." *Hastings Center Report* 26, no. 2: 30–37.

———. 1997. *Fragmentation and Consensus: Communitarian and Casuist Bioethics.* Washington, DC: Georgetown University Press.

Kuczewski, Mark G., and Patrick McCruden. 2001. "Informed Consent: Does It Take a Village? The Problem of Truth Telling and Culture." *Cambridge Quarterly of Healthcare Ethics* 10, no. 1: 34–46. Reprinted in part in *Taking Sides: Clashing Views on Controversial Bioethical Issues*, edited by Carol Levine, 14th edition. New York: McGraw-Hill, 2011.

Lidz, Charles W., Paul S. Appelbaum, and Alan Meisel. 1988. "Two Models of Implementing Informed Consent." *Archives of Internal Medicine* 148: 1385–89.

Mallon, William K. 2001. "Is It Acceptable to Discharge a Heroin User with an Intravenous Line to Complete His Antibiotic Therapy for Cellulitis at Home Under a Nurse's Supervision?" *Western Journal of Medicine* 174, no. 3: 157. www.ncbi.nlm.nih.gov/pmc/articles /PMC1071292/.

Mandava, Amulya, Christine Pace, Benjamin Campbell, Ezekiel Emanuel, and Christine Grady. 2012. "The Quality of Informed Consent: Mapping the Landscape: A Review of Empirical Data from Developing and Developed Countries." *Journal of Medical Ethics* 38: 356–65.

Nelson, Hilde L., and James L. Nelson. 1995. *The Patient in the Family: An Ethic of Medicine and Families.* New York: Routledge.

President's Commission for the Study of Ethical Problems in Medicine and Biomedical and Behavioral Research. 1982. *Making Health Care Decisions.* Washington, DC: US Government Printing Office.

Tice, Alan D., Susan J. Rehm, Joseph R. Daloviso, John S. Bradley, Lawrence P. Martinelli, Donald R. Graham, R. Brooks Gainer, Mark J. Kunkel, Robert W. Yancey, and David N. Williams. 2004. "IDSA Guidelines: Practice Guidelines for Outpatient Parenteral Antimicrobial Therapy." *Clinical Infectious Diseases* 38: 1651–72.

Wasson, Katherine, Mark Kuczewski, Michael P. McCarthy, Kayhan Parsi, Emily E. Anderson, and Paul Hutchison. 2017. "Navigating Clinical Ethics: Using Real Case Constellations to Guide Learners and Teachers in Medicine." *Southern Medical Journal* 110, no. 3: 195–99.

SECTION II

END-OF-LIFE
DECISION MAKING

Case 8:
The Stroke Case—
"I Can't Be Responsible for
Killing Your Mother"

SKILL BUILDER CASE: This case is designed for building clinical ethics consultation skills through simulation. Visit the ACES website for a video enacting this consultation and skills assessment materials at LUC.edu/ethicsconsult/.

Key Terms: *Durable Power of Attorney for Health Care, Palliative Care, Respect for Autonomy, Surrogate Decision Making*

Narrative

The patient, Mrs. Henderson, is a seventy-eight-year-old female. She was admitted to an outside hospital, where she was intubated before transfer for airway protection and was thought to have had a stroke. She was transferred to Big Teaching Hospital Medical Center (BTHMC) a day later, secondary to the possibility of surgical management of her cerebrovascular accident. At BTHMC, the patient was diagnosed as having had a significant right-sided ischemic stroke. The patient's husband is deceased, and her daughter, Patti, is an emergency room nurse. Before her recent stroke, Mrs. Henderson was a very active, independent individual, who was caring for her sister-in-law who had a stroke many years ago. Mrs. Henderson always said that she would not want to have things "dragged out like that."

When the patient arrived at BTHMC, the neurosurgeon determined that surgery would not help her. Currently, she is minimally responsive to pain, is ventilated, and is partially breathing above the ventilator, but is otherwise noncommunicative. Dr. Murphy, the neurologist, agreed that surgery was not an option and indicated that it would be several days before they could determine what her recovery would be like.

A family meeting was scheduled to discuss these findings with Mrs. Henderson's daughter, Patti. Because Dr. Murphy believed that it was clearly too soon to know if this patient would wake up or how severe the brain injury was, he asked to continue treatment for several days. Patty disagreed with Dr. Murphy's assessment of this situation and asked that all life-sustaining treatment be withdrawn. Given the impasse and possible values conflict, Dr. Murphy requests an ethics consultation.

Perspectives for Role Players

Dr. Murphy (a neurologist) [played by a physician in the video—an actor can be substituted]:

- You are not a big fan of withdrawing treatment altogether, but some cases strike you as worse than others. This case is one of the worst ones.
- You are very guarded about Mrs. Henderson's prognosis, and you feel that because it is an ischemic stroke (as opposed to a hemorrhagic stroke), she may actually improve to the point of regaining consciousness. You feel that to withdraw all interventions at this point would go against "standard of care" and could be considered "killing" the patient.

- Suggested phrase: "I don't want to / can't be responsible for killing your mother."
- Because this stroke is not in her dominant hemisphere, if she were to improve, she might actually be able to communicate.
- Of course, this stroke could progress, and she could possibly die.
- You would like at least five to seven days to see which way this goes. At that point she might not be on a ventilator even if she does not regain consciousness.
- Patti's insistence on withdrawal does not make any sense to you, because this patient just arrived here. After all, why was she transferred to BTHMC if treatment withdrawal was the goal?

Patti (the patient's daughter) [played by an actor]:

- You are rather sure of your mother's wishes because you talked to her all that time she cared for her sister-in-law post stroke.
- *Note:* Your mother has *not* completed a document giving you durable power of attorney for her health care and lists you as her agent. Her wishes have been expressed to you, her daughter, verbally but not in written form.
- You agreed to transfer her here to BTHMC because they said they might have an operation that would make her better. But, because they said surgery will not help, you would like to stop everything.
- During your health care education and experience as a nurse, you have seen many cases like this one, and know any additional measures are likely to be futile and may continue your mother's suffering.
- You feel some of the burden of carrying out your mother's wishes not to end up being "a vegetable" and dependent, but you are clear what she told you.

- You are not unreasonable. If they can definitely tell you when they will know if she will get better, then you will wait. But you want to know what the plan is if she does not get better—that is, what is the plan for allowing her to die?

Ethics Consultant [played by you]:

This case is tricky for a number of reasons that you want to explore in the ethics consultation:

- The patient has *not* completed a durable-power-of-attorney-for-health-care document. Her wishes have been expressed to her daughter verbally but not in written form.
- You want to respect the patient's wishes. But the context of the case makes you wonder whether a decision to withdraw life support at this point is premature and ethically inappropriate.
- You definitely think a couple of days of observation might be in order. But you want to pin the physician down on exactly when we will know something and what will happen then.
- You might want to mention a palliative care consult or hospice consult if the patient does not improve.

Ethical Analysis

In examining the issues in this case, one of the primary ethical considerations is to determine the patient's wishes. The gold standard in any case is to ascertain these wishes from the patient himself or herself whenever possible. The ethical principle supporting this standard is respect for autonomy. Western society places a high value on allowing individuals to determine what they want or do not want in a health care setting. Individuals with capacity can consent to or refuse treatments and interventions. In this case, Mrs. Henderson is unconscious and, therefore, unable to articulate her wishes. The ethics consultant must determine who the appropriate surrogate decision maker is, which will vary by state. Some states provide a specific order of surrogates, while other states indicate that the "next of kin" should make such decisions on behalf of the patient.

Here, Patti is the appropriate surrogate because Mr. Henderson is deceased and there are no other adult children. The role of the surrogate involves substituted judgment, meaning that Patti should speak as if she is Mrs. Henderson, and not simply give her own views or wishes.

A common ethical issue is how to weigh the benefits and burdens of different interventions. Currently, Dr. Murphy views the medical interventions as providing only benefits to Mrs. Henderson because they are allowing her the chance to recover. He is likely on the very conservative end of the spectrum in how he sees the situation. Many of his colleagues might consider the stroke to be fairly devastating and significant recovery to be more unlikely than he is portraying. Patti views the interventions differently; she believes that even if likely, partial improvement would not be of benefit to her mother because she would not want to be dependent. If she were dependent, her quality of life would be significantly diminished. The possibility of partial recovery is a greater burden in Patti's mind than it is a benefit. Helping the parties to articulate these views, explaining the underlying ethical norms and parameters, and offering ways forward are all part of the role of the ethics consultant.

Because Patti is the appropriate surrogate, Dr. Murphy needs to recognize her as such. The ethics consultant then needs to consider what views Patti is expressing on Mrs. Henderson's behalf. Patti indicates that her mother would not want to "live like this"—that is, in a diminished and dependent state. Dr. Murphy is strongly advocating for waiting five to seven days, which he states is normal—that is, the standard of care—for a stroke patient of this type, to see whether Mrs. Henderson improves as the swelling in her brain may decrease. Patti's concern is that her mother was clear about her wishes, and she worries that Mrs. Henderson will end up in a dependent state with a long recovery. She claims that her mother would not want this outcome and that respecting her autonomy means withdrawing life-sustaining treatment.

The differences in perspectives and values raise a classic dilemma for the ethics consultant—namely, trying to determine how a patient would react in this specific situation and the choices he or she would make in this context. The ethics consultant needs to facilitate a solution or way forward, which may entail a compromise on both sides, provided it is an ethically acceptable option.

Options could include:

1. Withdraw life-sustaining treatments, as Patti is requesting, and allow Mrs. Henderson to die (which respects the patient's autonomy, as articulated by her surrogate decision maker).
2. Wait five to seven days and reevaluate Mrs. Henderson's condition, and determine whether to continue aggressive measures or not. This is sometimes referred to as a "timed trial." In other words, Dr. Murphy could explain that the "standard of care" in cases like this is to wait five to seven days to see if Mrs. Henderson will regain consciousness. If she does, then she could be asked what her preference is regarding treatment. Waiting does not imply continuing with treatment; rather, the goal here is to clarify Mrs. Henderson's prognosis. If, after five days, the patient's condition does not improve, then the option of discontinuing treatment will again be discussed.

3. Compromise and assess the patient in three to five days, and then reconvene to make a decision.
4. Any decision to wait could include a discussion of placing a DNR order in the patient's chart. If she were to arrest, the medical team would not attempt resuscitation and would let "nature takes its course."

Case 9:
Futility—
"But She Said She Wanted Everything"

SKILL BUILDER CASE: This case is designed for building clinical ethics consultation skills through simulation. Visit the ACES website for a video enacting this consultation and skills assessment materials at LUC.edu/ethicsconsult/.

Key Terms: *Advance Directives (Oral), Surrogate Decision Making, Futile Medical Treatment, Potentially Inappropriate Interventions (or Treatments or Care)*

Narrative

Mrs. Czarniwicz is a sixty-seven-year-old woman who was diagnosed with nonresectable colon cancer six months ago. When that diagnosis was made, it was clear that the patient would eventually die, but it was not clear exactly when. The current admission to the hospital is the most recent of several admissions from a nearby nursing home for episodes of sepsis (infection) believed to be secondary to the entrance of bacteria through the friable colon cancer. On admission, the patient's general health appeared to be poor. Mrs. Czarniwicz looked emaciated, with generalized edema (swelling) and skin excoriation (abrasions). She could not move her legs and had only gross motor movement of her upper extremities secondary to severe spinal disease. She communicated mainly by head movements, such as nodding.

The patient was given antibiotics and steroids for treatment of the sepsis and made a "full code," based on discussions with her. She said that she wished to be resuscitated should the need arise. Three days after admission, Mrs. Czarniwicz developed acute shortness of breath, and a chest X-ray led to a differential diagnosis of congestive heart failure versus a pulmonary embolism. Mrs. Czarniwicz also developed acute gastrointestinal bleeding, believed to be secondary to the colon cancer. Over the next few days, diagnostic tests gave no additional insight into the patient's condition, and Mrs. Czarniwicz continued to become lethargic and confused. The lethargy could be accounted for in several ways, including possible brain metastases from the cancer. Her oxygenation was poor. Thus, she was intubated and admitted to the intensive care unit.

Mrs. Czarniwicz also developed a pleural effusion, and further malignancy is now suspected. She is septic, and pneumonia is thought to be the likely culprit. Her daughter, Sarah, has been asked what the medical team should do; and she, like her mother upon admission, requested that "everything be done."

Over the past few days, aggressive vasopressor therapy was begun to try and offset Mrs. Czarniwicz's dropping blood pressure. Nevertheless, her pressure has continued to drop, and ranged between 30 to 40 systolic on maximum vasopressor therapy. Over the next twenty-four hours, Mrs. Czarniwicz has become anuric and has developed massive generalized edema. She is oozing serous fluid from her skin and other puncture sites. Dr. Murphy called the ethics consultation service for assistance.

Section II

Perspectives for Role Players

Dr. Murphy [played by a physician or actor]:

- This patient is dying, and you feel compelled to make sure her daughter understands this fact.
- You plan to be quite blunt in your communication with Sarah to get her to accept how sick her mother is now.
- You would like to stop all aggressive treatment at this point, and are disturbed that the patient's daughter is asking the medical team to "do everything."
- You are not optimistic that Sarah will accept her mother's condition or agree to withdraw interventions.
- Ideally, you would like to stop the vasopressors, and if the patient arrests (which is likely to happen within a day or two) would prefer not to code her. That is, you want to enter a do-not-resuscitate (DNR) order.
- You are treating the sepsis and do not feel strongly one way or another about continuing the antibiotics (although you would rather stop them).
- You do not want to extubate the patient, because she would die very quickly afterward, and it would feel (and appear to the daughter) as if you "killed" her, even though you know that is not accurate ethically.
- Suggested phrase: "If we do everything you are asking, we will be 'torturing' / causing suffering for your mother."
- Suggested phrase: "What you are asking for is futile treatment."

Sarah Czarniwicz (the patient's daughter) [played by an actor]:

- You know that your mother is very ill, but believe that she could improve as she has done during each past admission.

- You realize that your mother will eventually succumb to the colon cancer, though you do not think this admission is that time.
- You want to give your mother every chance to recover.
- Suggested phrase: "She is a fighter."
- When first admitted, your mother stated she wanted everything done, including resuscitation.
- You are frustrated that the team keeps pressuring you when they know what your mother said she wanted when she was admitted.
- Conversely, you do not want your mother to suffer any more than is necessary if there is absolutely no hope of recovery.
- When there is no hope, you do not want the team to do anything that is painful for your mother, but you think that she should probably receive the interventions that do not hurt her—for example, medications, food, and water. You do not understand why the team would recommend stopping these interventions.
- Suggested phrase: "You just want to give up on her."

Ethics Consultant [played by you]:

- This hospital has no explicit futility policy.
- There is a statement in a policy on forgoing life-sustaining treatment that says physicians are not obligated to provide futile treatment. But the hospital's preferred approach is clearly consensus decision making in cooperation with the family.
- You want to make sure the words "death" and "dying" are introduced in this conversation, to ensure that Sarah is clear about the severity of her mother's condition. It is important to get the physician to say he believes the patient will die soon and certainly will not survive this admission.

- Then you want to shift the conversation to consider changing the goal of care from "prolonging the dying process" to "making the patient comfortable."
- If worse comes to worst, you will have to decide if you need to limit your goal to simply getting the surrogate to agree to a DNR order.

Ethical Analysis

Given that Mrs. Czarniwicz is intubated and not able to speak for herself, it is important for the ethics consultant to establish the appropriate surrogate decision maker. Sarah is the only child, and her father is no longer alive, leaving her as the appropriate surrogate. The ethics consultant should focus on determining what the patient would want and whether she has expressed her wishes in written or oral form. These questions highlight the importance of respecting the patient's autonomy and ability to make choices about her health care. Once again, the surrogate decision maker is the one to speak on the patient's behalf and represent her wishes because the patient does not have that capacity and is intubated.

One challenge in this case is that Mrs. Czarniwicz told the medical team that she wanted "everything done" when she was admitted a few days ago. Beyond wanting resuscitation, further content of that discussion with the team is unclear. Exploring what Mrs. Czarniwicz would want now, given her decline in health status and multiple organ failure, is a more nuanced conversation that illuminates benefits versus burdens, goals of care, and considerations about the quality of life (or death). The ethics consultant can help Sarah understand that when she is asked what her mother would want, she is not being asked to quote her mother's last utterance but to perform an act of "substituted judgment," in which she determines what her mother would likely say now, under the current circumstances.

The ethics consultant wants to ensure that Sarah understands the nature of her mother's current condition—namely, that she is dying. Having lived with the colon cancer diagnosis for six months, Sarah claims Mrs. Czarniwicz knew she would die eventually, but thought she would live for one year. She has been in and out of the hospital, and Sarah believes she will improve and be discharged as before. The concern of the physician is that Sarah is "in denial" about how ill her mother is and needs to hear the reality. The ethics consultant must try to remain neutral toward such assertions as she attempts to gather accurate and relevant information from all parties. A key piece of the ethical discussion and analysis will be the balance of the benefits and burdens of the current interventions. Sarah initially views the interventions as helping her mother, and Dr. Murphy sees many of them as burdensome for the patient. He is particularly concerned that Mrs. Czarniwicz will arrest and, without a DNR order, the team will need to attempt resuscitation, which will not be successful and will be harmful. And given her edema and skin condition, such an attempt will be very unpleasant, even distressing, for the code team. As she is actively dying, Dr. Murphy would like to withdraw multiple interventions that are not benefiting and are harming the patient.

The ethics consultant may need to introduce the language of death and dying if the physician or other health care professionals are not able or willing to do so. In this case, the physician is clear about the patient's deteriorating condition and that she is dying. Helping the surrogate decision maker absorb this new reality can be a key part of the ethics consultation process. Eliciting the patient and surrogate's views, given this new information, is important and can move the consultation forward as new goals of care discussions emerge. Shifting from a cure to care framework may help.

In this case, one turning point in the ethics consultation occurs after Sarah, the surrogate, realizes that the medical team has been doing "everything" to help her mother and that the disease progression and multiorgan system failure means that her mother is dying. She begins to focus on the harm and suffering caused, and her view shifts to try to avoid them. After that point, the ethics consultant is able to discuss ethically acceptable options with both parties. They agree to enter a DNR order for the patient to spare her from a resuscitation attempt if she arrests and to meet again in the next one or two days to review the goals of care again.

Case 10:
Withdrawing Treatment—
Easier Said Than Done

Key Terms: *Decision-Making Capacity, Forgoing Treatment, Suicide, Ethics Committees, Ethics Consultation*

Narrative

The patient, Mrs. M, was a fifty-four-year-old woman who was transferred to this tertiary care hospital's critical care unit from an outlying community hospital with a principal diagnosis of an acute anterior wall myocardial infarction—that is, a heart attack. Secondary diagnoses were acute pancreatitis, disseminated intravascular coagulation, acute respiratory failure, acute renal failure, and lactic acidosis. The patient was placed on a ventilator. Due to medication and her increasing medical problems, she was only periodically alert, but she was responsive when directly addressed. There were no written advance directives.

Mrs. M was hospitalized several years ago for acute pancreatitis. She also had a psychiatric history of anxiety and depression, and she had been consistently treated with Haldol and Prozac for several years. Mrs. M attempted suicide about ten years ago.

Her family consists of a supportive husband (Mr. M), an adult daughter (Martha), the daughter's husband, and a fifteen-year-old granddaughter (Rachel). The Ms have a son (Jake), who lived in the Midwest. He was not present at the hospital. Jake also had a history of depression and suicide attempts. The family informed him of his mother's serious condition, but they purposely kept him out of the decision making, fearing that he would act out if he saw his mother fulfilling his possible latent wish of wanting to die. Mr. M and Martha consistently voiced agreement that Mrs. M should make her own decision regarding treatment or a terminal wean. Mr. M said that his wife and he had talked about potential end-of-life situations. She was clear that she did not want to be kept alive if it would mean living in a more debilitated state or if the quality of her life would be compromised more than it already had been.

During her first three days of hospitalization, the patient was consistently aware and responsive. She was presented with the options of pancreatic surgery or drug treatments to relieve her excruciating pancreatitis. She was told that surgery had a high risk of mortality, with less than a 50 percent chance that she would survive the operation. Recovery would require extensive respiratory care, with possible placement for a period of time in an extended care facility, where she would be in a program for the redevelopment of skills for activities of daily living. Within these first three days, it also became clear that she would need to have dialysis. Mrs. M declined more medical intervention and expressed a desire to discontinue ventilator support.

With Mrs. M's decision, and the support of her husband and daughter, the attending physician agreed to a terminal wean. In a further phone conversation with the daughter on the day before the scheduled wean (the fourth day of hospitalization), the attending physician hesitated on the matter and called an ethics consult. The physician was concerned about Mrs. M's age and her potential to rally medically. The attending physician thought that treatment should clearly be "futile" before it was stopped, and he was not sure that it was presently the case. He was also concerned about Mrs. M's past history and her ongoing treatment for depression. He wondered whether her decision might be a kind of physician-assisted suicide. He also began to question the patient's decision-making capacity.

At this point, Mr. M and Martha became angry and distraught about the seeming reversal and the calling of "more people"—that is, the ethics consultation service. The husband and daughter had already communicated to Mrs. M that her decision was to be honored. They were also initiating their own anticipatory grief process before this apparent delay and potential reversal. The ambivalence in decision making moved this process into conflict and indecisiveness.

The Language and Issues of the Case

Once again, we have questions regarding the decision-making capacity of a conscious patient. But this time, any real questions about her capacity will be based on an alleged psychiatric disorder rather than cognitive deficits. To some degree, we see a struggle taking place about the label to be applied to this decision of the patient—that is, is it better labeled "suicide" or "forgoing treatment"? It is this struggle that seems to be raising questions in the mind of the physician concerning whether it will be a violation of his professional integrity to comply with the patient's wishes. As we have heard from his conversation with the patient's daughter, he believes that the appropriate label for this action is a function not only of the patient's intent but also the relative "futility" of the treatment being declined. Some specific questions this physician may need to answer include:

1. Should the patient's wishes and decisions be taken at face value without psychiatric evaluation? Should the severity of her medical condition automatically cast doubt on her decision-making capacity?

2. Should the physician abide by the wishes of the patient even if he has medical and ethical concerns, or should he have transferred care to another physician who had fewer problems with the situation?
3. What does "futility" mean in a case like this?
4. Whose decision is this? Does the patient's family's support for a position such as this one add to its moral acceptability?
5. Can an ethics consultation that is called by the attending physician be refused by the patient and family?

Perspectives and Key Points of View

Mrs. M: Throughout her hospitalization, she consistently communicated that she wanted no treatment to prolong her life. She wanted to be weaned off the ventilator. Living a sedentary life with increasing limitations on what she might be able to do or enjoy did not appeal to Mrs. M. She was a voracious reader, and limitations on such sedate activities were more than she could bear. Her family described her as no longer in love with life as such, but as "tolerating" it.

Mr. M (husband): He loved his wife, and even though he did not want to lose her, he maintained that her right to make her own decision was primary. He recounted their conversations about end-of-her-life decisions, in which Mrs. M was clearly opposed to an unnecessary prolongation of her life, even with a small medical possibility of recovery. Mr. M maintained two principal values, to which the whole family also steadfastly ascribed: promise keeping and not lying. He made a promise to abide by her wishes. He did not want to see himself or be seen as lying. Mr. M feared that the delay, caused by the physician, threatened to make it appear to Mrs. M that he was withholding the truth from her and not carrying out her wishes. Promising to abide by his wife's wishes and decisions had a higher value than maintaining her life, even with a low potential recovery.

Martha (daughter): She loved her mother, and even though there were some unresolved mother/daughter issues, she held to the values her father and mother espoused. She was adamant in supporting her mother's decision, and she resented the questioning of her mother's competency. She wanted to honor her mother and get on with the anticipatory grief process, to be with her mother in her dying. She, like her father, was hostile toward the physician and ethics consultant for delaying and potentially reversing what appeared to be an agreed-on decision.

The attending physician: He had second thoughts. He knew that the potential for long-term survival was low. Although the multiple consultations were in conflict about which organs might recover, the overall medical picture was bleak. Nevertheless, he was concerned that treatment still had benefit for this patient, and he feared that limiting treatment might be physician-assisted suicide, because the patient could be acting on suicidal thoughts emanating from an affective disorder. He raised competency issues, and then he became more ethically unsure of the decision.

Nursing staff: Nursing was continuing to provide good care. The patient's nurses clearly supported the patient and family. They were becoming irritated with the physician's and consultants' "part-versus-whole" approach to medical care and the delay in carrying out the patient's decision.

What Actually Happened

The chaplain had been in conversation with the family, the patient, and the attending physician. On the fourth day of hospitalization, there appeared to be agreement among all to meet the following morning to exchange views and review the decision. Instead, the following morning, the attending physician called an ethics consultation. The chaplain (who is an ethics committee member) and the on-call ethics consult team (a subcommittee of the ethics committee) met with the physician and eventually with the family. The ethics committee consultants (a party of four—two social workers and two physicians) reviewed the chart, the patient/family history, and the conversational tradition. The medical director of the critical care unit was brought in to address the issues of medical futility and comfort care measures in a terminal wean.

A meeting of all the people mentioned above and the family took place, in which the following were discussed and decided:

1. Competency appeared to be a moot issue. If the patient was declared incompetent, the husband and family would become surrogate decision makers. Because they were in agreement with the patient's decision, the decision to withdraw treatment would stand.
2. The issue of suicide was considered moot because the patient had not voiced suicidal ideation or exhibited acute depression before hospitalization and had consistently complied with antidepressant medication.
3. The family members reiterated their total agreement with the patient's decision.
4. The withdrawal of aggressive care process and the initiation of comfort care administration began, and the patient died within an hour, with her family at her bedside.

Case 11:
The Letter and Spirit of a Directive—
Making Decisions with a Patient
of Variable Capacity

Key Terms: *Advance Directives, Surrogate Decision Making, Ordinary Care, Forgoing Nutrition and Hydration*

Narrative

An eighty-three-year-old woman, Ms. U, was admitted to the hospital from an assisted living environment due to a stroke with left-sided weakness and aphasia. She had a history of Parkinson's disease, coronary artery disease, and a prior stroke several years ago. The day after her admission, she was seen by a neurologist, who noted dysarthria (i.e., problems of speech articulation due to muscular control disturbance) and a severely diminished gag reflex, and that she was not ambulatory. She did respond to right-sided commands. Speech and physical therapy were recommended.

A speech therapist also recommended that Ms. U not ingest anything by mouth, due to her swallowing difficulties. A Dophoff tube (a nasogastric tube) was inserted for feedings. Ms. U subsequently pulled out the tube twice; the neurologist's notes indicated that to survive, she would need a percutaneous endoscopic gastrostomy (PEG) tube, which is inserted into the stomach. At that time, her daughter, June, who lived nearby, refused the PEG tube but eventually agreed to a reinsertion of the nasogastric tube as a temporary measure.

The social worker spoke at length with June, who was initially reluctant to agree to any feeding tube at all because she wanted to follow her mother's wishes as expressed in her advance directive. This living will was one of the typical forms that are used in Pennsylvania. It was so worded that Ms. U did not want artificial nutrition and hydration if she were in a terminal condition or was permanently unconscious. The next day, June was still uncertain and was advised to confer with her sister, Donna, who lived out of town. It was hoped they would clarify their mother's intent. Ms. U's family physician also spoke with June and told her that a PEG tube was not an "extraordinary measure."

Due to uncertainty about the patient's decision-making capacity, a psychiatrist was consulted. He felt the patient was disoriented, lacked insight, had impairments of cognition, and was not competent to make decisions at that time. The social worker again spoke with June. June had spoken with Donna, and they were both in agreement to refuse any type of tube feeding.

During the next two days, Ms. U was seen again by the psychiatrist, who found her mental status to have gradually improved to the point where she appeared to understand what a PEG tube was and that it was necessary to provide her nourishment. He therefore found her to have the capacity for decision making at that time.

The hospital's ethics review group (the institution's "ethics mechanism") was summoned to review the case. It was determined that the living will was not applicable at this time, and therefore could not be honored. A decision was made that members of the group would contact Ms. U's daughters to address this issue. A conference call was set up for the next morning. After the new information was presented to June and Donna, they differed on the correct decision. Time was given them so that they could speak with each other without the review group present.

In the meantime, the patient was given a barium swallow. It showed that it was still not safe for her to take nutrition orally. Due to the psychiatrist's evaluation of the patient's decision-making capacity, he referred her for a surgical consultation. The patient thought she wanted a PEG tube but indicated that she wanted family agreement. Mrs. U's daughters were again contacted with this information, and they were presented with three options: (1) placing a Dophoff tube and physical restraints, to prevent the patient from removing it; (2) placing a PEG tube with no restraints; or (3) transferring their mother to another facility for evaluation and treatment. Shortly thereafter, June, who had voiced opposition to artificial feeding in the conference call, called the social worker to say that she agreed to the insertion of the PEG tube.

The Language and Issues of the Case

As is so often the situation, the questions in this case revolve around what it means to respect the autonomy of the patient. The patient has some ability to communicate, but it is not clear whether she is representing her wishes and values or whether the ethics review group is more or less eliciting the answers they are seeking. Thus capacity as well as the role of the family is at issue when a patient has questionable capacity. The family's interpretation of the patient's wishes displeased the treatment team, and precedence of interpretation is at issue.

This case squarely raises the question of whether a surrogate can make decisions for a patient in the same manner as the patient or whether the surrogate's latitude should be more restricted regarding what he or she may choose for the patient.

Perspectives and Key Points of View

Physicians and hospital staff: Both the attending physician and consulting physicians believed that it would be unconscionable not to "feed" the patient, because she was not terminally ill. The stroke left the patient with a diminished gag reflex, but it need not be life threatening.

The patient's daughters: Both daughters wanted to honor their mother's expressed wishes and to allow her a dignified death. They initially agreed, but then disagreed, on how best to honor these wishes in the current situation.

The patient: Ms. U had expressed in her advance directive that she did not want certain treatments if she was in a terminal state. According to the attending physician and the psychiatrist, she also seemed to express a desire to live at various points in this process.

What Actually Happened

The PEG tube was inserted about two hours after June's call. Within a few days, the patient was stable and was transferred to a skilled nursing facility. Several weeks later, the ethics review group received an emotional letter from Donna. The letter showed that she was feeling guilt about her concurrence with the treatment decision. In order to help Donna understand the advance directive and the informed consent process, the social worker wrote a letter to her reviewing the decision-making process in detail. There has been no further contact from the family.

Case 12:
How Competent Does
a Surrogate Need to Be?
A Decision Maker Who Might Not
Appreciate the Choice to Be Made

Key Terms: *Noncompliance, Surrogate Decision Making, Competence*

Narrative

A forty-nine-year-old woman, Mrs. Z, was admitted to Saint Anthony's Hospital due to cardiac arrest. She was intubated and placed on a ventilator in the emergency room. Mrs. Z's history is significant for two prior cardiac arrests, which were related to obstructive pulmonary disease and, secondarily, to heavy smoking, congestive heart failure, diabetes, obesity, hypothyroidism, and previous episodes of pneumonia. She had a long history of noncompliance with treatment plans, and she had continued to smoke until this most recent admission. Mrs. Z is a widow and lives with her daughter, son-in-law, and grandchildren. Her daughter and grandchildren are all believed to have mild cognitive impairments or developmental disabilities.

After ten days on a ventilator, the attending physician suspected Mrs. Z to be brain-dead. However, a neurological consultation and an electroencephalogram revealed some minimal brain activity. Nevertheless, the patient's chances of regaining consciousness or of returning to a high quality of life seemed minimal. Given this poor prognosis, there were two treatment options. First, a skilled nursing facility that accepts ventilator-dependent patients could be sought. Or life-sustaining treatment could be limited or withdrawn, and the disease process would quickly run its course. For instance, the patient could be extubated, and it was expected that she would die fairly soon thereafter.

The patient's daughter, Nora, was approached with these options. Nora was unenthusiastic about the prospect of a nursing facility, and she decided, after several days, that her mother should be extubated. A final meeting with the entire health care team was held to review this course of action, and all parties agreed on the plan.

The following day, Mrs. Z was extubated, but she continued to breathe on her own. She was transferred from the intensive care unit to a general medicine unit. The hospital social worker met with Nora to discuss nursing home placement. Nora, however, said that she thought her mother was going to die, and did not want to explore the nursing home options.

The Language and the Issues of the Case

The problem of the mental capacity of the surrogate decision maker clearly had the attention of the hospital staff. Thus, they are likely to discuss this case in terms of decision-making capacity. This raises issues including:

1. What should the team do if the patient continues to breathe for an indefinite period and is no longer appropriate for

the acute care environment, but the patient's daughter will make no discharge plan?

2. Is the patient's daughter competent to be the surrogate decision maker and this is a mere disagreement, or is it indicative of a larger capacity issue? If the latter, what action might be appropriate?

3. Is the hospital staff being less patient with the patient's daughter than they would be with other surrogates because of her perceived cognitive impairment?

Perspectives and Key Points of View

The patient's daughter (Nora): We have little insight into her thought processes beyond what we know from the recounting of the case. We know she believed her mother would soon die. It is not clear whether this was from a failure to appreciate the possibilities facing her or because she was relying on statements made by the physicians before Mrs. Z's extubation.

The hospital social worker: This social worker knew from experience that patients often do not follow the most likely medical scenario. That is, before extubation, it seemed likely that Mrs. Z would die shortly after the removal of mechanical ventilation. However, many patients, like this one, continue to breathe on their own for quite a long time. Because the patient would no longer be receiving any of the high-technology care that requires hospitalization, the social worker believed that the patient should be moved to another facility. The social worker also knew that a variety of institutional pressures would soon come to bear to make discharge of the patient imminent.

The social worker wished to avoid being too judgmental of Nora. However, from the social worker's point of view, Mrs. Z's care plan would be much simpler and could be handled more expediently if some other guardian were appointed.

What Actually Happened

No follow-up information on this case is available.

Case 13:
How Does a POLST Form Help?
When a Surrogate Contradicts
a Valid DNR Order

Key Terms: *Advance Directives, Competence, Decision-Making Capacity, Physician Orders for Life-Sustaining Treatment (POLST), Prehospital DNR Orders*

Narrative

Mr. M, an eighty-one-year-old man, presented at the Emergency Department of this hospital. During dinner at the nursing home where he lived, he had a fainting spell. The staff at that facility noted that he had poor color and low blood pressure following this episode and called an ambulance. He had coronary bypass surgery three years before and was believed to have Alzheimer's disease. Mr. M's wife was deceased, and he had one daughter, who lived nearby. She was very protective and concerned regarding her father. She communicates regularly with the nursing home. Mr. M was met by his daughter upon his arrival in the Emergency Department, and she remained with him.

Mr. M's medical records were sent with him from the nursing home, and they included a validly completed Illinois form for a physician order for life-sustaining treatment (POLST). The POLST indicated that the patient wished his care to focus on comfort, and it had been signed by a physician. This form was scanned into the hospital's electronic medical record in the advance directives section, and an entry calling it to the attention of the attending physician was made in the progress notes section of the chart, as per the policy of this hospital.

At 10:30 pm, Mr. M was admitted to a general medical/surgical unit from the emergency room. He was placed in a vest restraint at the request of his daughter, due to his past history of intermittent bouts of night-time confusion. However, at this time, Mr. M was oriented to time and place.

About a half hour later, a nursing assessment was performed on Mr. M. It revealed him to have a dusky color and abnormal lung sounds. His chest X-ray confirmed a diagnosis of pulmonary edema (the accumulation of fluids in the lung). Respiratory care staff were notified to perform a breathing treatment to increase the patient's lung expansion and improve his ability to breathe. About one hour after admission to the medical/surgical unit, the patient's daughter came to the nursing desk and stated, "My father is having difficulty." The nurse accompanied her to the patient's bedside and was unable to obtain Mr. M's vital signs. The nurse turned to the daughter and asked if she wanted her father resuscitated. The daughter said yes. A code was called, and a team responded with a crash cart.

The Language and Issues of the Case

Once again, the issue is what Mr. M would want and what processes maximize the opportunity to follow his wishes. Terms like "patient autonomy" are not particularly useful. Instead, we should ask certain questions:

1. What role should the POLST form play? It is a signed physician order. Of course, it was signed by a physician who is not on staff at this hospital.
2. What role should the family have in interpreting the wishes of the patient, given that he has a POLST? His daughter's consent to resuscitation seems contrary to the wishes of the patient, as expressed in the POLST and as ordered by the signing physician. Does the daughter's contemporaneous consent trump the documented wishes of the patient?
3. Did the patient have the capacity to make decisions at the time of the creation of the POLST form? Is this a question that the staff at the hospital should raise?
4. Was the way that the POLST form was handled at the hospital adequate? If not, how should the process be improved?

Perspectives and Key Points of View

The nurse: She was not sure whether it would be best to resuscitate this patient. However, given that there is no DNR order entered in the patient's hospital chart by a member of the hospital's medical staff, the nurse felt that she was obligated to call a code unless the patient's daughter refused it.

The patient's daughter: She thought her father "had suffered enough." She had watched the Alzheimer's disease progress, and she hoped that when death finally came, it might be painless and easy for him. It is still not entirely clear to the staff why the daughter did not refuse resuscitation. As best as she could relate afterward, at that moment it felt as if declining the code would be killing her father; the responsibility seemed overwhelming, and if they were offering resuscitation despite the POLST form, it seemed that it must make some sense to accept it.

The patient: We do not know what he thought. He seems to have been presumed to lack capacity on admission, despite being oriented to time and place. Of course, it is extremely likely, based on his POLST form, that he would have wished to decline resuscitation.

What Actually Happened

The patient was unresponsive to the resuscitation attempt. After approximately twenty minutes, the code was stopped and the patient was pronounced dead.

Case 14:
Withdrawing Treatment and the Family's "Returning Hero"— When One Family Member Says "Go" but the Surrogate Says "No"

Key Terms: *Surrogate Decision Making, Substituted Judgment, Patient Autonomy, Family Autonomy*

Narrative

The patient, Mrs. A, is a seventy-two-year-old woman with Alzheimer's disease. She was transferred from a nursing home to this acute care facility because of multisystem organ failure, including congestive heart failure and impaired renal function. She also had a urinary tract infection secondary to serratia, a bacteria associated with opportunistic infections. The patient had a long medical history and was well known at this hospital.

Mrs. A's history was significant for ongoing hypertension and a pulmonary embolism ten years earlier. After this embolism, the patient had a number of cardiac and pulmonary complications, which had contributed to a rapid progression of the Alzheimer's. Two years before the current admission, Mrs. A suffered a brain stem stroke with "locked in" syndrome. She was intubated, and a gastrostomy tube was inserted. She was able to understand spoken and written words. She was hospitalized for an extended period (several months) and was eventually transferred to a nursing home. Physical therapists saw little, if any, rehabilitation potential in the patient.

Mrs. A had lived with her husband until the stroke two years ago. Mr. A had his own health problems. He was an insulin-dependent diabetic with an amputation above the left knee. Because of his physical challenges, Mr. A realized that he could not take care of his wife and consented to the nursing home placement. He was quite upset by this state of affairs, but he seemed rational in discussing the treatment issues and the appropriate course of action. A son from San Francisco, Jeremy, also arrived at the hospital and told the attending physician and staff that all decisions should come through him, because his father and mother were "obviously no longer capable of handling these things." Jeremy concurred that nursing home placement was appropriate and should be initiated.

The current hospital admission was approximately two years after that placement episode. Mrs. A was still ventilator dependent, and her mental status had deteriorated over the course of the year to the point where a preliminary diagnosis of a persistent vegetative state was made. The husband was grief stricken and agreed with the attending physician that limitations of aggressive treatment seemed appropriate. Nevertheless, Mr. A wished to speak with his minister regarding what his religion had to say on the matter. After two conferences with his minister and the hospital chaplain, Mr. A agreed that a DNR order should be entered on the chart. He also began to favor withdrawal of the respirator, although a final decision had not been reached when the attending physician received a call from Jeremy's attorney. The attorney stated that treatment should not be limited in any way until Jeremy arrived in town and reviewed the situation.

When Jeremy arrived, he was accompanied by his wife, who was seven months pregnant. Jeremy wished his mother to be kept alive until his wife delivered the baby, so that his mother could "see" her grandchild." Mr. A believed that Jeremy had "taken leave of his senses," because Mrs. A could not "see" anything, and to prolong her indignities for two additional months would serve no purpose. Nevertheless, the fear of Jeremy bringing a lawsuit temporarily froze the decision-making process.

The Language and Issues of the Case

This case initially calls to mind all the usual terminology of end-of-life cases that we have explored in this section. We find ourselves thinking about how to respect the patient's autonomy and wondering about what role her son's wishes have in this situation. We can clarify this scenario by asking two basic questions:

1. Who is the appropriate decision maker for Mrs. A?
2. Is Jeremy's request to delay withdrawal of treatment for his social goal (letting his mother "see" the baby) a legitimate request?

Perspectives and Key Points of View

Jeremy: It is hard to attribute a single definitive motive to him because his motivations appear to shift on the basis of different considerations. In the hospital's earlier encounter with Jeremy, he focused on making sure that his mother got all the care she might need and that the physicians paid attention to her needs. He needed to be reassured of this fact before concurring with the nursing home placement. During the current crisis, his motivation seems to have shifted to a particular social goal—that is, symbolically linking this birth and death in his family. No matter what the motivation, he seemed determined to play an important role in the decision-making process.

Mr. A: Mr. A was well liked by the health care team. He was dutiful toward his wife and concerned about her well-being. He had never been very fond of Jeremy and disliked his son's domineering style. Mr. A was not very patient with Jeremy, and this resulted in little direct communication between them. In the initial case conference, Mr. A seldom addressed Jeremy directly.

The attending physician: He wished to see that the right thing was done, but he had grave concerns about trying to keep this patient alive for an additional sixty days or so. He believed that administering cardiopulmonary resuscitation (CPR) if she arrested or doing other invasive treatments, if necessary, would be contrary to "what is good for her."

The nursing staff: They were very impressed with Mr. A and liked him a great deal. Jeremy's personal style, which was domineering and controlling, was offensive to them, and they wished to protect Mr. and Mrs. A from his "craziness."

What Actually Happened

The attending physician contacted the hospital's legal counsel. The lawyer told the physician that this decision could legally be made by Mr. A in concert with the physician. However, much trouble could be avoided if they could get Jeremy to concur.

After two days of conferences with Jeremy, he agreed with his father's decision to withdraw the respirator.

Case 15:
"They're Crazy!"
The Micromanaging Family

Key Terms: *Surrogate Decision Making, Competence, Potentially Inappropriate Care*

Narrative

The patient, Mrs. O, is a fifty-five-year-old woman with metastatic colon cancer. The attending physician and treating team are clear that they believe that the patient is "actively dying." She is unconscious most of the time, but according to the patient's family members and some reports from members of the medical team, recently she has had an occasional moment or two of relative lucidity. Her two adult daughters, who spend most of the day at her bedside, report that these moments are few and each day are rapidly becoming fewer. The patient also has a husband and adult son, who visit for a couple of hours each day.

The plan of hospital care is, in some ways, relatively clear. The patient's husband is clearly the appropriate surrogate decision maker when the patient is unable to speak for herself, and in initial discussions, he agreed with the attending physician that comfort care was to be pursued and that the team should no longer attempt to cure the patient's cancer. There is a DNR order in the patient's chart. There had been some deliberation about appropriate placement—for example, whether the patient should remain where she was in the hospital and be comforted until her death ensues, placed in an in-patient hospice bed, or be discharged to her home, with hospice care if possible. Given her prognosis of only a very short time to live and the difficulty in transferring her out of the hospital, an in-patient hospice bed would be ideal. Unfortunately, the patient's insurer declined to authorize in-patient hospice care, thereby eliminating that option.

Of particular concern is that the patient's husband and son have idiosyncratic ideas about the patient's condition and care, and they have expressed them in a confrontational manner. For instance, the patient's husband asserted that he did not believe that the patient's abdominal discomfort was caused by metastases but by an echinococcosis infection, and he wanted treatment for it. Later, as the patient lost interest in food, the patient's husband and son wanted albumin given to her so that "she would get strong enough to eat" (i.e., they believed she was not eating because she was not strong enough to do so). So the physicians found themselves consistently trying to fend off requests for tests and treatments that were not indicated. At times, these refusals greatly frustrated the husband and son, who would then suggest that they wanted the goals changed to life extension if they could not get their way. The attending physician called for an ethics consultation.

The Language and Issues of the Case

This scenario is increasingly common, although it seems to have no name. That is, surrogate decision makers who have idiosyncratic theories and seek to micromanage portions of the patient's bedside care seem to be becoming more commonplace and an increasing motivator of requests for ethics consultations. As in this case, the overall treatment of the patient may be proceeding in a reasonable direction, but the constant confrontation and negotiations with family members can be quite taxing for the treating team. Some questions that might help clarify the situation include:

1. To what extent do we know the patient's wishes, and how? Is it possible to speak with her during moments of lucidity? Can what we determine regarding her wishes be used to help guide further conversations with the family?
2. Does the family have any hidden concerns, such as a fear of caring for the patient at home during her dying process?
3. Do all members of the family share these unusual views? Is it possible to meet with the entire family to clarify the treatment situation?

Perspectives and Key Points of View

The patient's adult daughters: They are well liked by the treating team because they are at the bedside constantly and are mostly concerned with their mother's comfort. They express annoyance with their father and brother's desires to try various approaches to their mother's illness. However, they are not very confrontational with their father and brother when they disagree.

The patient's husband: We know what he says, but we do not have a fuller picture of his motivations or worldview.

The attending physician: She wishes to keep the patient as comfortable as possible until the patient dies or is transferred to a more appropriate placement. The physician is frustrated by the family members' requests for treatments that will not help the patient and the amount of time taken up by the daily discussions with the patient's husband. She takes the time to explain everything to the family, including why many of the things they request are not indicated. On a few occasions, she has acquiesced to running tests for various infections, as requested.

What Actually Happened

The ethics consultant supported the attending physician in declining to provide treatments or tests that are not consistent with the plan of comfort care or that have no realistic hope of benefiting the patient. He also offered to help speak with the family.

The attending physician remained very patient in her conversations with the patient's husband and son. When they threatened to change the goals of care, the attending physician simply explained that she had nothing further that would foster the patient's life extension or cure the patient. Thus, changing the goal would lead to little difference in the patient's care. Two days after the ethics consultant was first called, the patient died comfortably.

Practical Commentary and Tips on End-of-Life Decision Making, with a Cheat Sheet for Dealing with Cases 8 through 15

Most clinical ethics consultation services still report that end-of-life decisions are involved in the majority of their consultations. This is somewhat surprising, owing to the fact that such decision-making processes have been developing for several decades and many facilities have medicalized this process through palliative care consultation services. Nevertheless, clinical ethics consultation services continue to be engaged in cases involving end-of-life decisions for a variety of reasons, including that they can provide a nonmedicalized facilitative process that helps in clarifying values and perhaps even producing a consensus on how to proceed (Aulisio, Chaitin, and Arnold 2004; DuVal et al. 2001; Swetz et al. 2007; Wasson et al. 2016).

A few things are worth keeping in mind on a practical level. First, it is sometimes mistakenly thought that there are no longer cases in which the patient or surrogate wishes to forgo life-sustaining treatment and a physician believes that this decision has come too soon. Such cases still occasionally find their way to clinical ethics consultants. They require that the consultant establish a process at whose end, if the patient/surrogate still disagrees with the physician, physicians will nevertheless respect the patient's autonomy.

Second, more often, consultants encounter cases in which the patient or surrogate is asking for "potentially inappropriate" or futile treatment (Bosslet et al. 2015). In these cases, knowledge of institutional policy regarding the extent of unilateral physician decision making is required. Educating the parties so that institutional policy is transparent, as well as helping each party understand the perspective of the other and their values, are the bread and butter of ethics consultation. And, even with new and improved mechanisms, such as POLST forms for conveying a patient's wishes, methods of implementing those wishes continue to be a challenge. In the end, the clinical ethics consultant is sometimes the final means for surfacing a way of implementing those wishes.

The cheat sheet is as follows:

1. *Case 8:* The ethics consultant will face a very pragmatic issue. Namely, if common ground on a treatment plan cannot be found, how might the patient and her daughter access a physician who would likely be more amenable to their point of view? Dr. Murphy's position is probably more conservative than one a typical neurologist might take. The ethics consultant should probably formulate a strategy to help Patti access a second opinion, if needed. This might be done by raising the issue in the case conference and offering to request the opinion through the department chair or medical chief of staff. Additionally, a palliative care consultation could bring a palliative care physician's perspective to bear. The ethics consultant should consider which institutional structures are best to use in the service of a second opinion or if Patti wishes to go outside the institution for a second opinion.

2. *Case 9:* As noted in the "Ethical Analysis," the ethicist will need to help the surrogate decision maker to understand that we are not simply seeking the words of the patient but

also an interpretation of what the patient would likely choose, given the current fact pattern. The consultant is also well counseled to be transparent regarding how far the team is willing to honor the choices selected by the surrogate. That is, if the team is planning to invoke a futility or conscientious objection policy because they are unwilling to perform CPR in these circumstances, the ethics consultant should explain this unwillingness early in any conversation with the surrogate decision maker. Conversely, if the ethics consultant believes that the policies of the hospital require that the team perform resuscitation if the surrogate continues to request it, the consultant should explain this to the attending physician and the team. He or she should explain the values and reasoning behind such an approach and also offer resources—for example, chaplaincy, patient relations, and social work—to deal with any resulting distress.

3. *Case 10:* Clinical ethics consultants are often called long after the optimal time. As a result, their initial effectiveness can be impeded by the family's desire to not want to deal with "more people." In a case such as this, in which the patient's and her husband's wishes are relatively clear and it is their right to make this decision, the consultant's goal is not obvious. Perhaps it is to provide a review to ensure the quality of the decision-making process, in light of the patient's age and history of depression. In such a situation, the consultant might do well to reassure the patient and her husband that their wishes, as they are clarified through the review process, will be honored after the review process. This communication may defuse any defensiveness about further conversations, because they will understand that the consultant is not there to override their rights.

4. *Case 11:* The clinical ethics consultant might keep several things in mind. First, the patient seems to need the support

of her daughters to make a definitive decision. This consult should probably culminate in a discussion that includes the patient and her daughters. Second, trying to determine the realistic options for the patient will be helpful. If the patient does not have a feeding tube of some sort placed, oral feeding will likely result in the patient getting aspiration pneumonia sometime soon after discharge. How can she avoid being sent back to the hospital and then receive treatments she would not want, such as artificial nutrition and hydration? As a result, the clinical ethics consultant should explore the possibility of her being discharged to her home or to a nursing home with hospice care or, at minimum, identify an appropriate physician who would be willing to complete a POLST form or perhaps a durable power of attorney for health care. Having such options elaborated in advance will make possible a richer and more meaningful decision-making discussion with the patient and her daughters.

5. *Case 12:* At this point, it is important for the ethics consultant to help the team identify and list options rather than focus on the surrogate decision maker's capacity. It is morally respectful to presume capacity of adults, and we do not have much evidence that the surrogate's abilities are inadequate to the task at hand. Furthermore, it would simply be impractical to pursue the naming of a guardian. The ethics consultant should work with the social worker and any palliative care resource persons to determine if there is a more appropriate placement within the hospital, such as an in-patient hospice bed. The discussions with the patient's daughter might involve negotiations that respect her opinion that her mother might die soon but also require that if she is still doing well after a defined period, additional placement arrangements will be made.

6. *Case 13:* There was no ethics case consultation involved in this scenario. But clinical ethics consultants need to work with their institutions to have appropriate procedures for effectively utilizing patients' POLST forms. The fact that its meaning was not considered at the time of admission and that a DNR order was not entered in the hospital's electronic medical record is disappointing and problematic. Leaving the discussion of the POLST implementation until a crisis moment can result in ineffective decision making that fails to honor the patient's wishes. The ethics consultant may need to raise the wider issue with the Ethics Committee and hospital administration to address this issue in the future.

7. *Case 14:* This is a common type of a scenario, and the clinical ethics consultant can help facilitate a process that usually results in the newly arrived family member joining the consensus established by the family members who have been at the bedside and better understand the situation, both cognitively and affectively. The skills challenge for the consultant will be to convey the information to Jeremy early in the process that his father is the patient's surrogate decision maker and that Jeremy has no real decision-making rights for the patient. Such information is best delivered early, and also in a matter-of-fact way that is not meant as a challenge to his zeal. It might be best discussed in terms of the roles of family members as supporting and providing input to the main decision maker, the patient's spouse. Managing expectations can be an important role and contribution of the ethics consultant in such cases.

8. *Case 15:* It is not entirely clear how the clinical ethicist can be helpful in this situation. Providing reassurance to the physician and treating team that they need not provide requested treatments that are not medically indicated in any way for

this particular patient can potentially reduce the moral stress they may feel. It also enables them to negotiate with the family from a position of strength. Following up after the case is over to debrief may also reduce any residual stress that they feel and might enable a clinical ethics consultant to develop additional strategies based on experience.

Conceptual Framework

In general, a long-standing legal and ethics consensus guides end-of-life decision making (Meisel 1992, 2005). At the core of this consensus is the notion that the patient's wishes are the ultimate guide to decision making. The tradition of how to make decisions regarding forgoing treatment builds on the tradition of informed consent. That is, the patient's wishes are the "gold standard" when it comes to refusing treatment. If the patient has the capacity to make the decision to refuse treatment, then he or she may do so. Interventions by health care providers are meant to determine whether the patient actually possesses the capacity to make the decision and has a grasp on the situation. As was noted in the discussion of informed consent, the lengths to which the health care team or ethics consultants must go to ensure that the patient is truly decisional and appreciates the ramifications of his or her choice is often considered relative to the risks involved. By implication, many of the same problems that arise in implementing the informed consent process recur in making end-of-life decisions, especially when the patient lacks capacity. Nevertheless, the standards for decisions when the patient lacks capacity are also a part of the consensus.

Section II

In making decisions for patients who lack decision-making capacity, surrogate decision makers should apply, in serial order, any directives the patient has left, the substituted judgment standard, and the best interests standard. This legal jargon should not be off-putting. Because the patient's wishes are always the gold standard, when a patient is no longer able to give contemporaneous consent or refusal, we should ask (1) if the patient left any explicit directions regarding what he or she would want—that is, an advance directive. If not, we then ask (2) knowing everything the surrogate decision maker knows about the patient's values, what would the patient likely choose in the present situation? Only when both these possibilities fail—for example, if we are making a decision regarding an incapacitated "John Doe"—should we ask (3) considering the burdens and benefits of treatment for the patient, what decision is in the patient's best interests?

Clinicians and clinical ethicists need to be aware of these standards and assist families in understanding and applying the correct standard. Families initially may be resistant to withdrawing death-delaying technology, but when they are asked "What would your (father, mother, husband, wife) have wanted?" it is easier for them to make a decision that is different from what *they* (the family) may want. Families sometimes find it easier to say that their father would not have wanted these interventions than to say that they do not want him to have to live this way. Obviously, this is not always the case, but families may find it easier to decide what their loved one would have wanted than to make a decision based on their own desires and feelings, because the latter may seem as if they are devaluing his remaining life. It is important for the ethics consultant to remember that the surrogate (family) must live with their decisions on behalf of the patient. Sometimes, or often, the burden of decision making, especially at the end of life, is great and surrogates need support, guidance about their role, and time to make these decisions (even when the clinical team is frustrated and pressing for a decision).

In general, these decisions are best made at the bedside without recourse to the courts. The courts should be utilized only when there is an intractable conflict that cannot be resolved or adequately negotiated by the clinical ethics consultant and other caregivers, or when the patient needs additional procedural protections, such as the appointment of a guardian, because they lack anyone to make decisions in their interests.

Difficulties in Implementing the Consensus on Making End-of-Life Decisions

Things do not always work out in practice as easily as they do in theory. End-of-life care is certainly no different. Three typical problems include (1) difficulty determining the patient's preferences; (2) problems of communication between the providers and patient/family; and (3) psychological inhibitions, practice habits, and legal misunderstandings of the health care providers. Let us examine each of these in order.

Patients often vacillate regarding what they say they want. Patients typically get better at knowing what they want if they have experience with various treatments over the course of a long-term chronic illness. For instance, patients who have been placed on a mechanical ventilator for chronic pulmonary disease come to know whether they would be willing to receive ventilatory support and be weaned from it again in the future. Of course, many patients must make decisions about treatments with which they have no experience. They may have misconceptions from watching medical dramas on television—for example, they may falsely believe that CPR is usually effective, or have drawn erroneous inferences from classic cases in the news, such as those of Karen Ann Quinlan, Nancy Cruzan, and Terri Schiavo (Pence 2014); and they may not know that people are sometimes successfully weaned from a ventilator. As a result, the first step in this process is always to make sure that patients and/or their surrogates receive basic information about the proposed treatments and the prognosis with and without treatment. This information must be given in words that the patient and/or surrogate can readily understand. It is also important for a clinical ethicist to remember that patients and families may not "hear" everything said to them, and repetition may be required before a patient or surrogate understands. This can be frustrating, but it is common, and decision makers need to be given substantial deference in this regard. They need to absorb complex new information, usually at a time of high emotional distress. In this regard, three specific types of problems merit a closer analysis, as follows.

First, preferences are not always fixed. What patients say might sound like a preference, but may be a sentiment that is uninformed by actual experience of a treatment or a malady. Patients may repeat a preference often enough so that it sounds convincing, even when it is not stable.

The choosing of treatments at the end of life or the creation of advance directives must not be seen as a one-time event. Like informed consent, end-of-life decisions are best viewed as processes. The process is one in which the patient comes to understand what the physician is thinking and what the physician is looking for when she asks certain questions, and the patient's values and goals become transparent to the physician. In this process, the patient gains additional experience and knowledge of his or her illness and comes to know his or her treatment preferences.

Second, there may be communication problems. One such problem is that sometimes the health care provider does not offer enough prognostic information. Early in the course of diagnosis and treatment, physicians may be reluctant to definitively answer questions by patients and family members regarding the future of the patient. The physician might respond by saying things such as "It's too early to tell."

However, the physician's thinking is likely to evolve rather rapidly. By in-patient hospital standards, a few days are a long time. By patient and family standards, a few days are a very short time. When the physician then must approach the family and discuss terminating life-sustaining treatment, this may come as a surprise to the family and provoke a variety of reactions. These reactions should not necessarily be taken at face value, because the family may simply need time to process the information and deal with their grief.

Another communication problem is that the physician may ask questions without providing enough context for the patient or family to make a good decision. This kind of problem results from good intentions; that is, the physician wishes to respect the patient's autonomy. However, if family members are asked if they "want everything done," they will certainly reply affirmatively. Health care providers must provide some guidance regarding what patients and families normally do in such circumstances. It helps alleviate problems that result when families become uneasy and think that perhaps only hard-hearted families withdraw life-sustaining treatment from their loved ones. And, of course, there is simply the problem that when health care professionals ask open-ended questions, patients and families logically assume that any answer they give is acceptable (Why would you be asking them if they wanted something unless it was OK to say yes?). Offering a menu of options without some guidance makes it difficult for the family members to weigh the options or fully grasp the specific consequences for their loved one. Families often seek this guidance by asking the health care providers "What would you do if it was your mother/father/spouse?"

And still another communication problem is that mixed messages are transmitted by a variety of different health care providers to different family members, who each have their own interpretation of the situation. Diagnostic and prognostic information can change rather quickly—

especially in an acute care setting. A large number of professionals may be involved with the patient's care (some of whom may rotate on or off the service during the course of a patient's care), and it is natural for family members and friends of the patient to try to figure out what is happening. This kind of problem can often be resolved by a group meeting called by the health care team or an ethics consultant. In addition, selecting one point person for communication in particularly complex cases streamlines the information and promotes clarity. Of course, this approach may not be practical or available in every setting.

Third and finally, health care providers may have psychological inhibitions, practice habits, and legal misunderstandings. These types of problems work together. Medicine is a practice as well as a science. Practitioners can form habits in the ways they think about and do things. These can be hard to change. For instance, a physician may come to understand that it is ethically acceptable to forgo life-sustaining treatment yet may never have been mentored through supporting a patient with comfort care at the end of their life. As a result, the ethics consultant must provide more than verbal information and would benefit from the assistance of a palliative care consultation.

Furthermore, health care providers get used to forgoing life-sustaining treatments given certain conditions and certain medical indications and do not often offer it under other conditions and indications. When the wishes of patients and families depart from these standard choices, health care providers often wish to stand on a position that is based on the premise that "It is not medically indicated" and want this claim to trump the patient or family's decision. Although, in some circumstances, such justifications are adequate—that is, a treatment simply will not work—"medically indicated" cannot be a term that covers over value differences or unusual preferences if patient autonomy is to mean anything.

The Role of Surrogate Decision Makers

The role of surrogate decision makers is fairly clear from the exposition up to this point. Surrogates are meant to help us understand the patient's wishes. Patients sometimes encode their wishes in an advance directive, such as a living will, a durable power of attorney for health care, or a physician's order for life-sustaining treatment. Occasionally, these wishes may be developed in detail and given a degree of specificity that enables direct implementation without interpretation (a POLST may achieve this goal in the best situations). But patient wishes often need to be interpreted and applied to the situation at hand, and the surrogate (whether designated in the directive or a close family member) can be of help in this interpretive process. When such directives are not available, the surrogate must proceed based on his or her knowledge of the patient.

As we saw in the points of the legal consensus, the surrogate should proceed according to the substituted judgment standard of decision making. According to this standard, the surrogate takes everything he or she knows about the patient—that is, his or her values and preferences—and tries to choose as the patient would. In essence, the surrogate should attempt to answer the question "If the patient could sit up and tell us what she wants, what would she say?"

Because the patient's wishes are the gold standard, it is only when all these other standards have failed to produce an answer to treatment questions—for example, informed consent, advance directives, and substituted judgment—that we proceed to make a decision based on criteria other than the patient's wishes. When we know little about the patient—for example, we are treating the proverbial "Jane Doe"—we seek to determine what is in the patient's "best interests." Determining what is in the patient's best interests involves balancing the burdens of treatment—for example, pain and suffering, and violations of dignity—with the potential benefits of treatment. Because different people make such calculations differently, the best interests standard normally involves trying to balance these in a way that an ideal "reasonable person" might (Kopelman 2007).

Beyond the Consensus: "Futility" and Physician-Assisted Suicide

The consensus on how to make end of life decisions is, as noted above, built on informed consent. The paradigm cases, such as those of Karen Ann Quinlan and Nancy Cruzan, that applied the doctrine of informed consent to end-of-life decisions are of a certain form (Menikoff 2001). They presuppose a model in which the health care provider is proposing treatment and the patient is making a decision to accept or refuse that treatment. In the classic end-of-life cases, the physician was insisting on a treatment that the patient did not want. So, the considerations we have detailed are all means of assuring a high-quality process that supports the patient or surrogate decision maker in making an informed choice to accept or refuse treatments in accordance with their values and considered preferences. But as we have seen in this section, not every case fits that paradigm.

Many of the problems in the clinic involve situations in which this paradigm does not hold. That is, they tend to be problems related to the less clear positive rights to treatment—for instance, when patients and families demand treatment that the provider or community believes is inappropriate. Problems surrounding requests for potentially inappropriate treatment (futility) and physician-assisted suicide can be seen to follow this pattern. Can one request treatment that the physician does not believe will help (futility)? Can one request help in killing himself or herself (physician-assisted death, or aid-in-dying)?

Active euthanasia and assisted suicide (sometimes called by terms such as "aid-in-dying") have been treated in the United States as morally and legally distinct from forgoing life-sustaining treatment. It is important for health care practitioners to understand that our legal system (and many ethicists) separates forgoing treatment from assisting a patient with suicide. Withdrawing and withholding treatment are thought to be guaranteed by a patient's right of self-determination. States may pass laws that require much evidence that the patient wants to forgo treatment. But states cannot legislate away the right of patients to forgo treatment. States can, and most do, legislate against assisting in a suicide. Meanwhile, the practice of assisted suicide is legal and well established in Oregon and Washington; and a growing number of states, including California, now offer an assisted suicide option.

It is crucial for a clinical ethicist to understand this point. Families often need to be educated on the distinction between withholding or withdrawing medical support and causing death. Many ethicists agree with this distinction and are able to help and support families as they consider making a decision for their loved one. However, if an individual ethicist does not agree with this point, it is still important to explain to the family that these are legally and, in many traditions, morally distinct options. Families from religious backgrounds or from a more traditional social milieu will find forgoing treatment a plausible option but may recoil at the direct taking of life.

The term "futility" is invoked by health care professionals to indicate that they are talking about treatment that they believe does not make sense to provide based on some standard of evaluating the effect of treatment. As a result, they would like to be able to make the decision to withhold or withdraw treatment that is deemed to be futile without the permission of the patient or family. For this reason, this debate often focuses on "unilateral DNR orders"; that is, physicians sometimes desire to make the determination that cardiopulmonary resuscitation is futile and thereby not provide it. This desire emanates from the fact that families might request that "everything be done" if they are asked about forgoing life-sustaining treatment for their loved one.

In essence, the question is whether some treatments may pose so little benefit that physicians and health care providers may simply withhold treatment without a patient's or surrogate's permission. Of course, this requires that one knows what futility means. In the classic article on the topic, Stuart Youngner analyzed the concept as consisting of four categories:

1. Physiological futility: The treatment simply will not achieve its physiological aim; for example, CPR will not restart the heart.
2. Postponing death: The patient will soon die, despite the administration of treatment.
3. Quality-of-life futility: The patient may live for an extended period with treatment, but in a very diminished state.
4. Poor probability of efficacy: The treatment might accomplish its aim, but the chances are, at best, remote.

It is important to note that there is a reasonably broad-based consensus around the first definition. This means that if a treatment is physiologically futile—that is, it simply will not produce its intended effect—a health care professional has no clear moral obligation to provide it. For instance, if a patient requests antibiotics for a viral infection, it is difficult to claim that the physician has a moral obligation to write a prescription for the antibiotics. Similarly, if it is clear that CPR will not restart the patient's heart or that vasopressors will not maintain the patient's blood pressure, it seems to be uncontroversial that health care professionals should not provide them. (Of course, we know that for pragmatic reasons, physicians do sometimes indulge requests for such treatment, i.e., write prescriptions for antibiotics where they are unlikely to be useful.)

The doctrine of informed consent, which is the foundation of the consensus on forgoing life-sustaining treatment, speaks against using any kind of quality-of-life judgments as the basis for unilaterally forgoing life-sustaining treatment (Helft, Siegler, and Lantos 2000). The doctrine of informed consent is founded on the value of the self-determination of patients. Each patient gets to make his or her own judgment about the value of additional days, months, or years of life with an illness or disability. As a result, unilaterally making a determination to withhold CPR or other life-sustaining measures because the patient's resulting quality of life will "not be worth it" is a judgment that our ethic has difficulty countenancing.

Futility policies have proliferated over the years. They generally involve a process of conversations and reviews by medical staff to provide concurrence on the grave medical prognosis and projected inadequacy of additional treatments. They often require that the case be reviewed and discussions of the parties be facilitated by a clinical ethics consultant. The policy may support a unilateral determination with regard to a DNR order by the physicians, or it may simply end with the review process but leave the final determination of resuscitation or other care with the patient or surrogate decision maker. This process approach has recently been supported in a major interprofessional society's consensus statement on potentially inappropriate care (Bosslet et al. 2015). Because such treatments may distress caregivers, ethics consultations related to such care now form a large part of the requests for clinical ethics consultation. However, rather than making definitive pronouncements in favor of unilateral decision making by the health care team, clinical ethics consultants generally emphasize process, skillful communication, and support (Curtis et al. 2005).

References and Further Reading

Aulisio, Mark P., Elizabeth Chaitin, and Robert M. Arnold. 2004. "Ethics and Palliative Care Consultation in the Intensive Care Unit." *Critical Care Clinics* 20, no. 3: 505–23.

Berlinger, Nancy, Bruce Jennings, and Susan Wolf. 2013. *The Hastings Center Guidelines for Decisions on Life-Sustaining Treatment and Care Near the End of Life.* New York: Oxford University Press.

Bosslet, Gabriel T., Thaddeus M. Pope, Gordon D. Rubenfeld, Bernard Lo, Robert D. Truog, Cynda H. Rushton, J. Randall Curtis, Dee W. Ford, Molly Osborne, Cheryl Misak, David H. Au, Elie Azoulay, Baruch Brody, Brenda G. Fahy, Jesse B. Hall, Jozef Kesecioglu, Alexander A. Kon, Kathleen O. Lindell, and Douglas B. White, on Behalf of the American Thoracic Society's Ad Hoc Committee on Futile and Potentially Inappropriate Treatment. 2015. "Responding to Requests for Potentially Inappropriate Treatments in Intensive Care Units (An Official ATS/AACN/ACCP/ESICM/SCCM Policy Statement)." *American Journal of Respiratory and Critical Care Medicine* 191, no. 11: 1318–30.

Chung, Grace S., John D. Yoon, Kenneth A. Rasinski, and Farr A. Curlin. 2016. "US Physicians' Opinions about Distinctions between

Section II

Withdrawing and Withholding Life-Sustaining Treatment." *Journal of Religion and Health* 55: 1596–1606.

Curtis, J. Randall, Ruth A. Engelberg, Marjoiri D. Wenrich, Sarah E. Shannon, Patsy D. Treece, and Gordon D. Rubernfeld. 2005. "Missed Opportunities during Family Conferences about End-of-Life Care in the Intensive Care Unit." *Journal of Respiratory and Critical Care Medicine* 171: 844–49.

DuVal, Gordon, Leah Sartorius, Brian Clarridge, Gary Gensler, and Marion Danis. 2001. "What Triggers Requests for Ethics Consultations?" *Journal of Medical Ethics* 27, no. s1: i24–i29.

Helft, Paul R., Mark Siegler, and John Lantos. 2000. "The Rise and Fall of the Futility Movement." *New England Journal of Medicine* 343: 293–96.

Kopelman, Loretta. 2007. "The Best Interests Standard for Incompetent or Incapacitated Persons of All Ages." *Journal of Law, Medicine and Ethics* 35, no. 1: 187–96.

Meisel, Alan. 1992. "The Legal Consensus about Forgoing Life-Sustaining Treatment: Its Status and Its Prospects." *Kennedy Institute of Ethics Journal* 2, no. 4: 309–45.

———. 2005. "The Role of Litigation in End of Life Care: A Reappraisal." *Hastings Center Special Report* 35, no. 6: S31–S36.

Menikoff, Jerry. 2001. *Law and Bioethics: An Introduction.* Washington, DC: Georgetown University Press.

Pence, Gregory. 2014. *Medical Ethics: Accounts of Ground-Breaking Cases,* 7th edition. New York: McGraw-Hill Education.

Swetz, Keith M., Mary Eliot Crowley, C. Christopher Hook, and Paul S. Mueller. 2007. "Report of 255 Clinical Ethics Consultations and Review of the Literature." *Mayo Clinical Proceedings* 82, no. 6: 686–91.

Wasson, Katherine, Emily Anderson, Erica Hagstrom, Michael McCarthy, Kayhan Parsi, and Mark Kuczewski. 2016. "What Ethical Issues Really Arise in Practice at an Academic Medical Center? A Quantitative and Qualitative Analysis of Clinical Ethics Consultations from 2008–2013." *HEC Forum* 28: 217–28.

Youngner, Stuart J. 1988. "Who Defines Futility?" *Journal of the American Medical Association* 260, no. 14: 2094–95.

Youngner, Stuart J., Robert M. Arnold, and Renie Shapiro. 1999. *The Definition of Death: Contemporary Controversies.* Baltimore: Johns Hopkins University Press.

SECTION III

DECISION MAKING FOR MINORS

Case 16:
"God Can Do Miracles, and He Will Heal Jessica"
A Pediatric Patient Wants to Forgo Treatment but Her Parent Disagrees

---

SKILL BUILDER CASE: This case is designed for building clinical ethics consultation skills through simulation. Visit the ACES website for a video enacting this consultation and skills assessment materials at LUC.edu/ethicsconsult/.

Key Terms: *Informed Consent, Assent, Futile Medical Treatment, Mature Minor, Potentially Inappropriate Interventions (or Treatments or Care)*

Narrative

Jessica Jones is a fourteen-year-old female who was diagnosed with acute myeloid leukemia (AML) three years ago. She had a stem cell transplant, multiple rounds of chemotherapy, and radiation therapy. She has been in remission, but the AML has now recurred. Her mother, Marissa Jones, is very involved, and accompanies Jessica to all her appointments and treatments. Her father died two years ago from a heart attack. Jessica has two younger siblings, ages ten and six. The family are devout Christians who strongly believe that God will heal Jessica. Their pastor has visited Jessica in the hospital on multiple occasions to pray for her healing and recovery. Jessica herself welcomes these visits and has talked openly about her faith.

Given the return of the AML, Jessica's oncologist, Dr. Cook, recommended a second stem cell transplant, which she received two weeks ago. Initially, it seemed that this treatment was working and that her AML was responding. But for the past week, the medical team has suspected that Jessica's condition is not improving and that her AML is advancing. Mrs. Jones has refused to engage in conversations about what might happen if this treatment does not work. She continues to stress that the AML went into remission before and will again. The nurses report that Jessica is very weary of the treatments and has begun to express to them that she does not want to continue. The nurses claim she understands what that would mean—that she would die—and she is prepared to accept that end. She openly states that she is a Christian who believes in heaven and is not afraid to die, though she does not want to leave her family or upset them. When the nurses tried to talk with Mrs. Jones about Jessica's views, she became agitated and stated, "Jessica doesn't know what she is saying. She doesn't really understand what it would mean to give up now," and "God can do miracles, and He will heal Jessica."

After multiple conversations with Mrs. Jones, the attending physician, Dr. Cook, requests an ethics consultation to try to address the situation. The ethics consultant gathers the relevant parties to discuss Jessica's current condition.

Perspectives for Role Players

Mrs. Jones (the patient's mother):

- You want to give your daughter every chance of recovering from her AML.

- You are not ready to accept that the stem cell transplant is not working, and you still hope that some experimental treatment might be effective.
- You are frustrated that the nurse is saying that Jessica does not want to continue her current treatment.
- You feel as if Dr. Cook and his team are "giving up" on Jessica.
- You are not ready to let Jessica go without exploring all the options, including obtaining a second opinion.

Dr. Cook (a physician who is an oncologist) [played by a physician or actor]:

- You are clear that the second stem cell transplant has not worked and that Jessica's disease is progressing.
- You do not believe that there are any other available treatment options that will cure her.
- You want Mrs. Jones to accept that Jessica is no longer in remission and is going to die.
- You are frustrated that Mrs. Jones continues to focus on other treatment options when, in your expertise, there are not any to be offered.
- You are an expert in the field and feel that Mrs. Jones does not trust your judgment.

Nurse [played by a nurse or actor]:

- You know that Jessica is dying.
- Jessica has told you that she desires to stop the treatment because of all the side effects.
- You have experience with patients like Jessica and are confident in your rapport.
- You understand the burden on the patient and want to help alleviate her symptoms.

- You want Mrs. Jones to hear what Jessica has said and give weight to this patient's decisions, even though she is a minor.

Ethics Consultant [played by you]:

- You want to understand the perspectives of both Mrs. Jones and Jessica.
- You will attempt to build a picture of Jessica's wishes (in absentia) and why the health care team thinks she wants to stop the treatment.
- You explore Jessica's role in the decision-making process and the various rationales for her role.
- Questions you want to explore in the discussion include: What weight should Jessica's views have in this process? Who will ultimately make the decisions about Jessica's medical treatment?
- You also want to foster a clear, common understanding of Jessica's prognosis.

Ethical Analysis

This case presents ethical issues and challenges that differ from those involving adults. Jessica is a minor (fourteen years old), so she does not have ultimate decision-making authority for herself or the same degree of autonomy as do adults over eighteen. Although she is old enough to have some insight into her AML, her mother has parental authority and is ultimately (ethically and legally) responsible for her well-being. Jessica's age and level of insight into her condition provide an area of potential conflict because she seems to be expressing a desire to stop the treatment, while her mother is adamant that the medical team continue to treat her. How much weight to give Jessica's wishes versus her mother's position is a key area of exploration for the ethics consultant. Standards for decision making for minors (i.e., persons under eighteen years of age) give the ultimate responsibility to the parents for most medical decisions.

Part of the ethical nuance in this case owes to Jessica's accumulated experience and knowledge of medical treatment. Because Jessica has been through a stem cell transplant, she has detailed knowledge of how she felt and coped. She expresses her weariness at feeling so bad and about her diminished quality of life. Ethical standards give more weight to the decisions of pediatric patients as they grow closer to being considered adults and gain capabilities. At fourteen, Jessica is still a child, but she seems to be a mature one, with much insight and high emotional intelligence for her age.

The nurse attempts at multiple points to have Mrs. Jones hear what Jessica has been telling the nurses—namely, that she is ready to stop the treatment because of her diminished quality of life and the burdens of an ineffective treatment. Jessica is not experiencing any benefits from this stem cell transplant, because it has failed. Some (including Dr. Cook) would consider this treatment to be "futile" because it is not producing remission, the desired physiological effect. Jessica is only experiencing the treatment's side effects and its burdens, including fatigue, nausea, and cachexia. She claims to be weary of the treatment, and she wants to stop it. She knows she will die if the treatment does not work, and thus she understands the consequences of her choice. Her faith is important to her, and her pastor and Christian community provide support. On one level, Mrs. Jones dismisses Jessica's conversations with the nurses, indicating that these must have taken place on "bad days." But on another level, Mrs. Jones wants Jessica to talk with her about these feelings. The ethics consultant suggests that talking with an adolescent psychologist might be helpful for both parties.

As the ethics consultation progresses, Mrs. Jones raises questions about the success of the current treatment, other treatment options, and experimental treatment trials. She is not prepared to withdraw all interventions from Jessica, and wants to pursue other options. She and the physician continue to disagree about options, and it becomes clear that a second opinion should be obtained in order for her to process Jessica's current condition and the recurrence of the AML. Mrs. Jones has lost some degree of trust in the medical team because she views the news that Jessica is dying as them "giving up" on her. Because her request is reasonable and ethically justifiable, the ethics consultant should help Mrs. Jones obtain a second opinion. If it had not been raised as an option, the ethics consultant could have offered it for Mrs. Jones to consider.

Ultimately, Mrs. Jones is responsible for the decisions made about Jessica's medical care and treatment. The challenge for the ethics consultant is to uphold this parental responsibility while also helping incorporate Jessica's wishes, as an insightful teenager, and that of the health care team members, who see the failed stem cell transplant as "futile" and thus as only producing burdens for the patient.

Case 17:
Transfusions as a Preventive Measure for a Witness Child— Do the Child's Medical Interests Outweigh Family Integrity?

Key Terms: *Autonomy, Decision-Making Capacity, Family Integrity, Religious Beliefs, Religious Values*

Narrative

RC is a thirteen-year-old girl who has sickle cell anemia. She first came to the children's hospital two years ago, after the family moved from their home in Chicago. She was diagnosed as having sickle cell anemia, also known as sickle cell disease (SCD), which is a genetic disorder that causes a patient's red blood cells to become stiff and sickle shaped. The disease causes a variety of symptoms, the most prominent of which is crises that are caused when the "sickled" cells block small capillaries, preventing the flow of oxygen to limbs and organs. This blockage is called sludging. The crises range from mild bone aches to debilitating body pain, infection, acute splenic crisis, aplastic crisis, acute chest syndrome, gall bladder stones, renal disease, and stroke. Currently, there is no cure for the disease. RC has had many hospitalizations for pain and fever crises, and her most recent hospital admission was for her first stroke episode.

RC is supported by her family—which includes her mother, her father, and her brother, who also has SCD. She is doing well in school, despite missing many days for her hospital admissions and clinic appointments. She and her family are devoted Jehovah's Witnesses, and they draw their community support from this group as well.

She has been seen in the pediatric hematology clinic for the past two years and has had her symptoms and pain crises managed in the hospital or in the outpatient infusion treatment center. Since her most recent hospitalization, she has had mild hemiparesis (paralysis on one side of the body) in her right hand; but she has felt that this is resolving since her discharge and with the aid of physical therapy. She is being seen in the pediatric hematology clinic for an evaluation and treatment plan regarding her most recent episode.

The pediatric hematologist has recommended that RC be treated with chronic blood transfusions to prevent future stroke episodes. Strokes occur in about 10 percent of children with SCD, and the risk of recurrence after a first stroke is even greater. The pediatric hematologist stated that an important stroke prevention clinical trial for such patients has shown that chronic transfusion therapy is highly effective in reducing the chance of stroke in high-risk children with SCD and may also help reduce acute chest syndrome and pain episodes.

The chronic transfusion treatment plan comes with risks of transfusion reaction, iron overload, and alloimmunization (an immune reaction to the blood cells). RC is considered at greater risk for another stroke due to her increase in frequency of admissions for pain crises and her recent stroke.

After a very long discussion with the family, the parents state that although they feel that the treatment of chronic blood transfusion would offer their daughter some benefit, they refuse it, based on their religious beliefs as Jehovah's Witnesses.

One week later, RC was admitted for an SCD pain crisis, and at that time her pediatric hematologist strongly recommended the chronic transfusion treatment plan. RC's family members and the pediatric hematologist had a conference, which also included the hematology/oncology social worker, primary inpatient nurse, outpatient clinic nurse, pediatric neurologist, and pediatrician. The treatment plan was discussed, but the family continued to refuse the blood transfusion treatment plan.

After consultation with the medical legal office, the pediatric hematologist sought a court order to override the parents' refusal and to treat RC with the chronic transfusion treatment in the best interest of RC.

The Language and Issues of the Case

The language of this case potentially could take two roads—that is, one could talk about parental choice and the role of religion in making choices for minors, or one could talk about the role of the physician and health care institution in acting in a minor's best interest. Of course, the parents' view and that of the physician are ultimately two differing interpretations of RC's best interests. Another way to discuss this case is also in terms of RC's possible decision-making capacity and her role in the choice. Although at thirteen years of age she would not able to make her own decision absent a court finding that she is mature enough to do so, we might consider whether that is worth exploring. If she is not the decision maker, how can we alleviate the stress that might result from being placed into a conflicting situation between her parents and her health care provider?

This case raises additional questions regarding the care and the autonomy of patient RC and her family:

1. Was the family's integrity respected? Is their role as RC's primary support system being appropriately addressed? Will they be well positioned to support RC if she develops complications related to the transfusions or if the chronic transfusion treatment does not benefit her?
2. How has the patient–family–health care provider relationship been affected by the decision that the pediatric hematologist has made to seek a court order to treat RC despite the family's refusal?

Perspectives and Key Points of View

The nursing staff: The nursing staff, both inpatient and outpatient, have developed a rapport with RC and her family from her many admissions and clinic visits. During her last hospitalization, the nurses were extremely concerned for the welfare of RC because her most recent crisis included a mild stroke that has left her with hemiparesis. The inpatient primary care nurse for RC has worked with other patients with SCD. She feels strongly that the treatment benefit of the chronic transfusion far outweighs any negative effects from compelling such a treatment, especially in a patient with RC's medical history.

Mrs. C: She is the mother of two children, both of whom have a chronic illness. She is very familiar with SCD because her brother's and sister's children also have it. She feels that she is close to her daughter and is very concerned about her welfare. RC's most recent admission has her scared because she has a niece who died as a result of an SCD crisis and a nephew who is now wheelchair bound as a result of a stroke from his SCD. Her son, who also has SCD, has done fairly well, without as many admissions as his sister.

She is very involved in her faith as a Jehovah's Witness and has drawn personal and family support from her faith. She does not question her faith's refusal of all blood transfusions. She states that she trusts God and his will to provide care for her daughter. Mrs. C has had a good rapport with the pediatric hematologist who has cared for their daughter. She has never questioned any treatment plan until now.

Mr. C: He is the quieter side of the family. He usually lets his wife do all the talking and decision making. He is there to provide financial and emotional support and discipline for the family, but he has left the medical decisions up to his wife.

He is also a practicing Jehovah's Witness, and he feels that his faith is what keeps him together, especially at times like this. The last admission for his daughter has him very concerned. However, the treatment of administering blood transfusions is something that goes against his faith, which he certainly does not want to do. What would the community think of him or his daughter if they let this happen?

RC: She is a very pleasant young woman who is well liked at her school. The last admission has left her with hemiparesis, causing a noticeable difference in her physical abilities, compared with her classmates. She is concerned that what happened to her cousin could happen to her—for example, she could become wheelchair bound. She states that she does not fully understand the "blood transfusion" issue, but she has been told that her faith will not allow it. She has stated that she feels caught between her parents' convictions and what the doctors want for her.

The pediatric hematologist: She has been taking care of RC for the last two years and has worked with SCD for most of her medical career of twenty years. She has seen many of her patients do well with the chronic transfusion treatment, and she feels that it may have prevented many admissions and possibly some strokes among her patients. She states that the clinical study data show that there is a documented reduced rate of acute chest syndrome in children who receive chronic transfusion compared with children who receive a transfusion only when indicated. Also, a major clinical trial has shown that chronic transfusions are highly effective in reducing the chance of a stroke in high-risk children with SCD. She feels that without the chronic blood transfusions administered as a preventive measure, RC will continue to have frequent admissions for pain and sepsis crises and will develop a devastating stroke in the future. Although she respects RC's parents' convictions as Jehovah's Witnesses, she feels that she needs to obtain the courts' intervention on behalf of RC so she can receive this treatment that would benefit her.

What Actually Happened

The pediatric hematologist was "successful" in obtaining a court order for RC to be treated with the chronic blood transfusions. The first transfusion was scheduled for the outpatient treatment center the following week. RC arrived via cab service. Her parents did not drive her to the hospital for treatment; nor was there any contact between the treatment center and her family. Information had to be conveyed through the social worker and a family friend. The first time RC received her transfusion, she was cooperative and quiet. She did not know quite what to expect. Subsequent transfusions became routine, aside from the lack of family involvement. One year passed, and at that time RC had reduced her hospital admissions from eight times the previous year to twice this year for pain and fever. Shortly after the year of treatment, RC and her family moved out of town and were lost to follow up. The relationship between the family and the health care providers was never quite the same. Her parents, who were previously involved in her care, did not always accompany her to her clinic visits, and they rarely visited her during her two admissions.

Case 18:
IV Drug Addiction and the Perfect Son— Difficult Decisions in Treating a Chronic Opioid User

---

Key Terms: *Autonomy, Decision-Making Capacity, Competence, Informed Consent, Surrogate Decision Making, Family Autonomy*

Narrative

W is a seventeen-year-old high school junior who was admitted to a community hospital with endocarditis. The clinical team quickly discovers that W has been injecting heroin for the past three months. This news comes as a surprise to his parents, who are clearly taken aback by it. The patient is an honors student, plays baseball for his high school, and has been scouted by several colleges for potential scholarship opportunities.

W admits to injecting heroin into his chest and other areas where needle marks would not be detected. The patient is started on a course of long-term intravenous (IV) antibiotics, and social services meets with the patient and his parents to discuss drug rehabilitation programs. The patient has an IV access port placed to receive his recommended six weeks of antibiotic therapy. His clinical status appears to decline, and he is observed to be lethargic and confused. Toxicology reveals that the patient has heroin in his system, and he admits that his visitors have been using the IV port to inject him. Visitation is restricted, but the team is extremely hesitant to discharge the patient to his home with home health care. W's parents both work during the day, and they cannot provide 24-hour supervision. He cannot go to a rehabilitation facility because of his medical needs, and he is refusing to stay in the hospital for six weeks. The attending physician calls the ethics consultation service. If this patient were an adult, the attending physician would inform the patient of his treatment recommendations and, assuming the patient continued to wish to leave, he would then pull the IV lines and allow the patient to leave against medical advice. Ethics is called because the physician does not know what his ethical obligations are in light of a minor patient's refusal to remain in the hospital.

The Language and Issues of the Case

This case raises questions concerning the standard of decision making to be used:

1. Should decisions be made for the patient in a paternalistic way, according to the best interest standard, because he is a minor?
2. Should the autonomy of this near-adult be respected, and should he be treated as a "mature minor" for the purposes of his treatment?
3. Practically speaking, because he is a large, athletic person, what can be done to help him if he decides not to cooperate? Forcing treatment on him for an extended period against his will does not seem to be a realistic option.
4. How does his addiction affect the plan of care?

Perspectives and Key Points of View

W's parents: Their sense of reality has been shaken to the core. They thought they had a dream family, and are stunned to discover their son is a heroin addict. Their image of such addicts does not fit with their situation. They now simply want to do anything necessary to get their son physically and emotionally well. But they no longer have any idea what to expect the future to be like.

W's physician: He wishes to know what his options and obligations are. He has generally had little success with people with substance use disorders, and hopes to be sure he does all the standard things that are required, even if he is ultimately unable to help the patient much.

W: He is deeply ambivalent. On one hand, he enjoys his "partying" and cannot imagine giving it up. Living in a hospital for six weeks seems like forever, especially if he cannot have any fun. On the other hand, he is deeply ashamed and cannot believe he has let his parents down to this extent. How could all this have happened after only a few months of "partying"? He wants to want to stop doing these things but has no idea how to acquire the desire to stop using heroin.

What Actually Happened

A nursing home was found that would accept the patient for the remaining four weeks of antibiotic therapy—if he signed a behavioral contract that included abstinence from using illicit drugs and enrolling in substance use counseling and treatment. One of the consulting physicians in the hospital was also on the staff of the nursing home. This connection facilitated the transfer, and this physician agreed to monitor the patient's progress. W was given a private room, but he had to participate in daily activities, eat in the dining room, and help other residents get around. The school district agreed to count his time doing these endeavors as community service hours.

W was allowed only family visitors and tutors from the school district. He became a very popular resident of the nursing home, and his outgoing personality returned. In particular, the older women residents and he interacted very amicably. He completed his therapy and was discharged to his home with his parents.

Case 19:
"She'll *Never* Be Able to Take Care of That Child!" Family Integrity and the Newborn's Best Interest

---

Key Terms: *Competence, Decision-Making Capacity, Family Integrity ("Treating the Family"), Best Interests Standard*

Narrative

Mrs. D was a forty-one-year-old woman, admitted after giving birth to a 4 pound, 7 ounce son in the ambulance en route to the hospital. The pregnancy was full term. However, Mrs. D did not know she was pregnant until her seventh month.

Mrs. D's medical history was significant for multiple sclerosis. She stopped taking her medications when she discovered that she was seven months pregnant. Mrs. D initially thought she was entering menopause, so she sought no further explanation of her missed menstrual periods. She had always adhered to her medical regimen, and stopped taking the medications on the advice of her physician. Before delivery, she had difficulty walking but was able to do so with the aid of crutches or by holding on to objects. She was independent in her activities of daily living, and she had been able to get around town because her husband could drive.

Mr. D also had multiple sclerosis. He reportedly was not as conscientious with his medical regimen as his wife. Although confined to a wheelchair, he was able to drive a car that had been modified to meet his particular needs. His driving enhanced the couple's ability to function independently in the community. Mr. D had a sister who lived in the area but with whom they maintained only minimal contact. There were no other nearby family members and no formal support systems. Mr. D, however, had been previously married, and he had a son from that marriage living in Texas.

In conversations with the nursing and social service staff members, Mrs. D indicated that she wished to take the baby home, but she requested assistance developing child care and parenting skills. She felt that she could manage with someone assisting her in her home three to four hours daily. Mr. D did not participate in any discussions regarding discharge planning needs but stated that he would agree to his wife's wishes. The couple's only source of income was a monthly Social Security disability payment, and they clearly would not be able to pay out-of-pocket for in-home services.

After giving birth, Mrs. D was hospitalized for three days. During her stay, the nursing staff raised concerns regarding her ability to care for her baby at home. Mrs. D's fine motor skills were poor, and on several occasions, the nursing staff believed that she would have dropped the baby if they had not been supervising the mother–infant interaction. At the urging of the nursing staff, the pediatrician decided that he would not discharge Baby D until 24-hour-a-day home health care was arranged.

The home care manager from the local visiting nurse association reviewed the situation and spoke with Mrs. D. He believed that the needs of the mother and infant were too great for them to meet. It was not possible for them to provide around-the-clock services. The county's child protective services agency was asked to evaluate the situation and make specific recommendations. The agency case worker made a home visit and subsequently met with both parents at the hospital to assess their ability to provide physical care for the infant. Mrs. D had been weakened by complications after delivery, so, due to her tremors, she required assistance getting in and out of a chair. Her coordination was poor, and she seemed incapable of placing and holding a bottle in a baby's mouth. Mr. D continued to be passive throughout the home visit, and did not put forward any personal preference about the outcome of the decision-making process but simply said, "Whatever," when asked for his opinion.

The child protective services agency decided to pursue temporary custody through the courts. Mr. and Mrs. D initially agreed with this plan, but then changed their minds. Mr. D's son in Texas was also willing to take the infant. During the next several days, Mr. and Mrs. D contacted an attorney and attempted to procure discharge of the child from the hospital.

The Language and Issues of the Case

The language of this case can take several turns. One can focus on Mr. and Mrs. D and speak about the rights of persons with disabilities and the discrimination that results from societal biases. Of course, the discussion can focus on the infant as the patient of the health care team members and emphasize their duty to look out for the child's interests. Or one can avoid terminologically pitting the interests of the parents against those of the child by seeing the family as a unit and talking about the health care providers' duty to "treat the family." Some questions worth exploring along each of these lines include:

1. Were the rights of the baby's mother adequately taken into account?
2. What was in the baby's best interests? What factors should be considered in addition to the parents' physical strength and dexterity?

3. Should more input have been elicited from Mr. D, or is this an issue that centers on the *two patients* (i.e., the baby and Mrs. D)?
4. Was the family's integrity respected? Who, ultimately, was in control—the hospital staff or the parents?
5. Should the attending physician have exerted a more pro-active approach in the discharge disposition of the mother and infant?
6. Were the roles played by the nursing staff and social services personnel appropriate?

Perspectives and Key Points of View

The nursing staff: The nursing staff were extremely concerned about the welfare of the infant, who was to enter what they felt to be a home with less-than-capable parents. It was clear that providing a safe environment in which the child would be cared for was a central concern, and the nursing staff did not think such an environment could be provided within the home. The nursing staff wished to be beneficent toward the infant and adopted an attitude of protective paternalism as their main value.

The social workers: This group was more sympathetic to the parents' need to have the infant in their care. The social workers solicited the involvement of the child protective services agency, originally with an eye to obtaining services to assist the parents in child care. The social workers, however, wavered in this commitment as the case progressed, and they were ready to go along with placement of the child.

Mr. D: His opinions were obscured by his reticence, and it was assumed that he was not the primary decision maker in the household.

Mrs. D: This mother bonded well with her child, and there was never any question of her mental and emotional fitness for motherhood. She believed that with a little outside help—that is, the three to four hours daily that she had requested—her physical challenges in caring for the child could be ameliorated. In fact, she thought that having the care of the child as a motivating force would help her to overcome the many daily obstacles of living with her illness. It was not clear at this time what she thought about her husband's role in this situation.

What Actually Happened

The judge refused to grant custody to the child protective services agency. Instead, he ordered the agency to provide 24-hour sitter service for thirty days until the home situation could be adequately evaluated. The baby was discharged to his parents, who took him home. Referrals were made to the federal Special Supplemental Nutrition Program for Women, Infants, and Children and to a program that screens children regarding developmental and educational needs.

For one year, the child continued to remain in the care of his parents, with in-home sitter services provided eight hours nightly. The mother was able to manage care during the remaining time. The child protective services agency continued to monitor the home situation. A year after the baby's discharge, Mr. D's physical health began to decline, and he was hospitalized some distance from the family home. During this period, Mrs. D and the baby went to live with her parents. Mr. D has subsequently made some progress in his recovery, and Mr. and Mrs. D are now divorced.

Case 20:
Families and Hope—
Fostering the Patient's Self-Determination

Key Terms: *Family in Medical Decision Making, Competence, Decision-Making Capacity, Do Not Resuscitate*

Narrative

RQ is a twenty-two-year-old divorced man with a diagnosis of end-stage multiple sclerosis. He has two living parents and one sister. The family dynamics are dysfunctional at best, stemming from events before the disease process was terminal. RQ had been living independently and had cared for his own medical needs until five years ago. As his disease progressed, he opted for an experimental drug therapy from Germany in hopes of a cure. His parents, Mr. and Mrs. Q, strongly favored this therapy, and they made their recommendation known to all involved. As his condition worsened, RQ had several hospitalizations and was cared for in his own home by his parents and home care agencies.

Because his parents had such strong personalities, RQ was often not included in decision making regarding his health care. This factor also made it difficult for home care staff and hospital caregivers to communicate effectively with the patient. Also, because the parents gave somewhat idiosyncratic directions and orders, the home care staff sometimes felt compromised in the care they delivered. There were ongoing conflicts throughout the entire time RQ was cared for at home. It seems that despite RQ's age, he had been sick for so long that he and his family have never moved beyond the parental and child roles. And as he had been cared for by the health system's pediatric rheumatologist for many years, he continued to be cared for by the Pediatrics Department during this advanced stage of his illness.

RQ and his parents constantly struggled among themselves for control over his care. The issue of where RQ should live was contested. He sometimes suggested that he should be alone, but his parents insisted that he live with them. During this time, RQ wished for independence, often fighting with Mr. Q and figuratively "throwing him out" of his room. However, the reality was that, at this late stage of his illness, it was impossible for RQ to care of himself, and he was dependent on his parents for help.

Early during the current hospitalization, RQ became critically ill with respiratory distress. He was quickly intubated and was transferred from the pediatrics floor to the intensive care unit. There, he was placed on a ventilator. He would indicate to staff that he "wanted the tube out," but the physician believed that this crisis was temporary and he had a chance of remission. So the physician and his parents thought his treatment should continue. No form of advance directive had been previously addressed, and no one raised the question of what to do if the patient's condition deteriorated. The attending physician did not approach RQ regarding these matters, because he thought that RQ was not competent to make such decisions. The consulting physicians did not know the patient well enough to participate in this discussion, and left this subject to the attending.

As the hospitalization continued, RQ became more and more agitated. So he was sedated and thereby became unable to voice his wishes. His medical condition deteriorated, and he eventually had a line inserted for hyperalimentation (nutrients), a tracheostomy tube placed, and was given a feeding tube. During this course, he had several bouts of infectious processes and Methicillin-resistant Staphylococcus aureus—known as MRSA—infection. As the hospitalization in the intensive care unit continued, RQ's father became more and more controlling of his care. He would forbid his wife or RQ to have discussions with the physician, pastoral care staff, social service staff, or hospital staff regarding future placement or the patient's code status.

As time progressed, RQ's condition stabilized. He was weaned off the ventilator. When the tracheostomy tube was plugged, RQ could speak. He initiated conversations with the staff. He said that he was ready to die, that he did not ever wish to be back on "that machine," and that he wanted to go home. His parents insisted that RQ be a full code and that all resuscitative measures be taken. The staff members became increasingly frustrated because they believed it was only a matter of time before he would need to be back on mechanical ventilation.

The Language and Issues of the Case

This case is prima facie one of conflict between a patient and his family members. Of course, as with many conflicts involving family members, the conflict takes place against a complex background of interdependency and care. The attending physician's assessment of RQ's decision-making capacity also placed it among the issues. This question of capacity will need to be settled in order to make progress in resolving the case. Specifically:

1. Does this patient have decision-making capacity in his present condition? If so, how should his right to self-determination be protected?

2. Just how far can RQ be "self-determining"? Can he make decisions regarding placement and disposition?
3. What are the rights of the parents as his caregivers? What are the duties of the health care team toward them? For example, can they deceive Mr. and Mrs. Q regarding code status if RQ so requests?
4. This family unit functions as if the patient is a minor, but he is an adult by the standards of the law. How should the ethics consultant approach this dynamic and the underlying legal and ethical considerations?
5. Should the health care team accept the family's way of proceeding, or does the team have an obligation to attempt to facilitate a transition to a more adult patient model of decision making?

Perspectives and Key Points of View

The nursing and social work staff: From their experience in caring for this patient for an extended period, they feel confident that they know he now has the capacity to make his own decisions. They believe he understands and appreciates that his condition is terminal.

The parents (Mr. and Mrs. Q): They have been caring for RQ for several years, and they believe they have the legal right to make his treatment decisions. They also feel he is not competent due to his illness and the effects of medication.

The physicians: RQ has a number of physicians caring for him, and they have expressed a variety of views over the course of his treatment. They are unhappy about the prospects of having to make a choice between whose wishes to honor, and they would very much like the patient and his parents to come to an agreement. Some physicians feel more strongly than others about where to draw a line in the negotiating process, but in general, they evince a wait-and-see attitude.

What Actually Happened

There were several multidisciplinary patient care conferences with the physicians, nurses, social service staff, administration, and others to discuss the patient's status and discharge planning. The attending physician consulted with a psychiatrist and told the family of the consult. But the attending physician neglected to mention that the purpose of this psychiatric consultation was to assess RQ's capacity to make his own decisions regarding do-not-resuscitate (DNR) status and other treatment choices. After full consultation and discussion between the attending physician, the psychiatrist, and the consulting physicians, a determination was made that this patient had capacity to make his own decisions.

The next morning, the attending physician signed an order form to limit life-sustaining treatment. When RQ's parents were informed, they were angry and hostile. They threatened to seek legal action and to remove the patient from the hospital. At this point, the hospital also sought legal advice and increased security to protect the patient from being taken from the hospital against medical advice, and also to protect the staff from any threat or risk from RQ's father.

After several days of talking with the patient and his family regarding the patient's wishes, the parents began to accept that RQ could make these decisions for himself. Sensing that positive developments were taking place, the hospital staff began to pursue discharge planning with the patient and family. Finally, after much education, planning, and care, RQ was discharged to his parents' home. He would be cared for by his parents and by home health care and other staff. His mother took a prehospital DNR form for use at home. When leaving the unit by ambulance, RQ thanked the hospital staff. RQ died at home, as he had wished, one week after discharge, with his father and mother at his side.

Case 21:
Who's the Patient?
Dealing with a Formidable Advocate

Key Terms: *Rehabilitation Ethics, Surrogate Decision Making for Minors, Best Interests Standard, Support Groups, Family in Medical Decision Making*

Narrative

JP was a four-year-old boy with spastic quadriplegia, secondary to cerebral palsy (CP). He was also delayed intellectually and functioned at an eighteen-month-old level. When JP was six months old, his developmental pediatrician referred him to a pediatric program at Saint Catherine's Rehabilitation Hospital for a comprehensive course of therapy—physical, occupational, speech, and hydrotherapy. JP was the fourth of four children. His sisters were seven, nine, and eleven years of age. There were no other significant medical issues or history in the family.

Over the course of the past three and a half years, JP and his parents had become quite interactive with the pediatric staff of the rehabilitation hospital. His mother and father took turns bringing him to therapy; they never brought him together. Once, JP's mother confided to the social worker that she thought their marriage was "on the rocks." She and her husband had wanted a son desperately, and when they found out about JP's developmental difficulties, things were never the same. Mrs. P felt she had failed as a wife, and she saw her main role as helping JP to be as normal as possible. She would do whatever she felt was necessary to achieve this end. She became active in local and state CP advocacy organizations, attended CP support groups, and was also quite active in her local school system. Mr. P was more passive; he watched JP's therapy and took instructions home, but he did not interact with JP any more than was necessary. Mr. P stated he loves his family, but it was hard for him to see his boy as a "helpless cripple."

From a therapeutic standpoint, JP's parents were able to understand and carry out a stretching/range-of-motion program, and they did an excellent job of maintaining this program. JP was able to stand with moderate support, and had been doing so for about six months. He was able to take a step or two in the pool with assistance, which has become a "crowning achievement" for Mrs. P. The speech therapist had been working with JP on swallowing. JP had a gastric tube for three years, and only recently had been able to attempt therapeutic feeds of pureed foods. Mrs. P stated that she had given JP solid food on occasion, and that he especially liked McDonald's french fries. She noticed that JP coughed sometimes when he tried them. However, she stated that tasting french fries and swimming are his only pleasures, and she does not feel the speech therapist should be taking one of these pleasures away from him. JP had one episode of aspiration pneumonia.

The treatment team had met by themselves, and they had also met with the physiatrist (a physician specializing in physical medicine and rehabilitation), who was the attending physician for the pediatric program. In their professional opinion, JP would probably never ambulate; and if he got to the point where he could take a step or two on dry land, it would probably be with much assistance and not functional or safe. They met with Mrs. P to tell her their opinion.

Mrs. P's response was to state that there were several mothers in her CP organizations whose doctors said the same thing about their kids. Mrs. P added that as long as she never gives up hope, he would walk. JP was to begin kindergarten in two months, where he would receive educationally based physical therapy, occupational therapy, and speech therapy. The therapy team felt that JP should be discharged from the pediatric program—except for speech therapy, to monitor his swallowing situation (a medical issue)—when he started kindergarten. The team thought that his other therapeutic needs would be met by his individual educational program in kindergarten. But when the physiatrist discussed this proposed termination of pediatric therapy with Mrs. P, she became quite angry and threatened to sue.

Mrs. P stated that JP's developmental pediatrician thought that this recommendation was "insane," and would write orders for JP to continue all therapies, especially the pool. Mrs. P said that she sees progress constantly, and that what the therapists were doing was helping him. She also believed that speech therapy is the least of his needs, and that he was ready to eat everything the family ate, except tough meat. The therapy team discussed this informally over lunch, and most of them thought that JP's mother was overly involved with him and in denial. The therapists felt compromised at the idea of being forced to continue therapy, even though they saw limited functional gains.

The Language and Issues of the Case

The language of the case will, to some degree, follow whichever issue one identifies as paramount. On one hand, there is the simple issue regarding informed consent. Although we usually focus on consent, its information aspect can be at issue. The treatment team believes that JP has reached a "plateau" and will not progress much further. But plateaus in rehabilitation can be somewhat subjective, and we do not know if the team members have adequately prepared Mrs. P to see that the plateau is impending and are accurately assessing the situation (e.g., should the information Mrs. P obtains at a support group be so easily dismissed?).

However, we can also choose to focus on the swallowing issue, which Mrs. P believes is a nonissue. JP has had a bout of aspiration pneumonia, which was probably attributable to these feedings. Is this event evidence that Mrs. P is not able to care for her child properly or is engaged in some form of child abuse? This situation raises additional questions:

1. What was the treatment contract? What did the professionals and Mrs. P agree to when they began treatment? In other words, what information was given, and when did consent occur? Has the process of informed consent continued? Have the treatment goals been revisited at appropriate intervals?
2. Is Mrs. P's ability to serve as a surrogate decision maker in question?
3. Are there child abuse/protection issues related to feeding JP? Should the staff of the rehabilitation hospital report this case to the local children and youth services agency?
4. Are there ethical conflicts among the professionals? That is, is there a conflict between the developmental pediatrician and the hospital staff that needs to be mediated?

Perspectives and Key Points of View

Mrs. P: Mrs. P is very adamant about the fact that JP still needs therapy as a medical treatment and that termination would do him and his family harm. She has educated herself through various special organizations and has been cooperative and compliant with all treatment and educational efforts up until this point, except for the recent feeding issues. When asked about the feeding concerns, Mrs. P states that the speech therapist is "a nice girl, but she doesn't know what she's talking about." Mrs. P says that JP does not cough that much when he eats at McDonald's, and that she knows cardiopulmonary resuscitation and the Heimlich maneuver if he does start to choke. Mrs. P states that she is willing to do whatever it takes to see JP continue in therapy, even if it means obtaining a lawyer. She says that the developmental pediatrician supports her point of view and also feels that JP needs to continue therapy.

Mr. P: He states that all medical and therapy decisions are Mrs. P's, and that he does not have much to say when it comes to JP.

The physiatrist: He believes that from a medical standpoint, JP's prognosis for functional walking is poor, yet he may be able to have a viable means of locomotion using a motorized wheelchair. He tried to approach this issue with Mrs. P, who refused to consider using a wheelchair as a treatment goal. The physiatrist believes that therapy at this point is maintenance; yet he acknowledges that "maintenance" is a gray area at best and that "in the old days" they would have kept JP in therapy, even at the maintenance level. The physiatrist is reluctant to disagree with the developmental pediatrician, but he states that therapy and mobility in his opinion have plateaued and that unless Mrs. P wanted to consider the use of a motorized chair in the future, and JP developed the skills needed to use the chair, JP's physical therapy, occupational therapy, and hydrotherapy should end. The physiatrist thinks that the only pertinent remaining medical issue is the feeding issue, which could be addressed with speech therapy. However, he said that Mrs. P is going to do what she wants, regardless of medical recommendations.

The therapists: They voice several concerns. They are concerned about Mrs. P because they have gotten to know her well over the past few years and have seen her exhaust herself on JP's behalf. The physical therapist and occupational therapist agree that they have done all they can to educate Mr. and Mrs. P with regard to JP's ongoing care. They believe that he has plateaued, so at this point the focus needs to shift toward the school and his "real life successes." The therapists emphasize that they are not recommending stopping all therapy but that therapy does need to shift to the educational setting, where JP's needs for occupational and physical therapy will be met.

The speech therapist is concerned that Mrs. P is in denial about the feeding concerns and that JP is at risk for aspiration and choking. The therapist voices frustration with Mrs. P and has taken numerous approaches to try to discuss these issues with her, and the therapist agrees that they are polarized and getting nowhere. She believes there will be progress in JP's ability to swallow safely, but it will take some time.

The social worker: She is concerned about the emotional status of the family and Mrs. P. The social worker thinks that marriage and family intervention around JP and the parents' experience of having a son with a disability would be beneficial to them emotionally. Improving their mental and emotional status might also help them to adhere to the new treatment regimen. However, there are no insurance funds available for this intervention, and the local Mental Health Department has a nine-month waiting list. In any event, Mrs. P is reluctant to try the Mental Health Department because of what she has heard in her advocacy groups. Mr. P states that he is willing to try, but he is concerned that Mrs. P would not get involved. The social worker is also concerned about the frustration of the team and their polarized position vis-à-vis Mrs. P. Because of the future risk of JP aspirating (due to Mrs. P's feeding attempts), the social worker wonders whether there is a child abuse issue here or the potential for one.

What Actually Happened

This team met again with Mr. and Mrs. P to review the recommendations and solicit their feedback. The team's agenda focused on concern about the feeding issue; the need to terminate physical therapy, occupational therapy, and hydrotherapy; and the switch to an educational focus. Mrs. P seemed to focus on concerns that she and JP were being abandoned and being told there was no hope. The team was able to reframe some of these concerns so that the "graduation" from the program was seen as a move forward, not backward. The team and the parents were able to contract for periodic reevaluations of JP's rehabilitation status—with the understanding that when JP is able and ready to benefit from more intervention, he would be considered for an outpatient program.

The physiatrist asked for and received permission to reinforce this plan with the pediatrician. The team also evaluated norm setting with parents of children entering the pediatric program and reevaluated this aspect of the program. The social worker was able to set up a brief intervention, focused on engaging Mr. P in JP's care, helping Mrs. P come to terms with her son's differences, and reestablishing them as a couple. Once this brief intervention was completed, the parents continued counseling at an outpatient mental health facility.

Practical Commentary and Tips on Decision Making for Minors, with a Cheat Sheet for Dealing with Cases 16 through 21

Cases in which the patient is a minor are often among the most difficult for clinical ethics consultants. In general, one wants to establish trust and a partnership with the patient's parents, guardians, and/or other key persons involved in making decisions for or with the patient. Parents are often quite naturally protective of the patient, so they can be defensive when they think their judgment might be being questioned. As a result, a clinical ethics consultant will often do well to allay suspicions by directly expressing and reiterating that he or she can see the parent's concern and care for their child. Making supportive statements acknowledging how difficult this situation must be for them and recognizing the expertise they have in understanding the patient can help establish a partnership. This partnership can be essential because the family usually must be involved in the implementation of the patient's long-term care plan for that plan to be effective.

When the patient may have some capacity to participate in the decision-making process, the clinical ethics consultant must be careful to try to help the patient's perspective to be heard but must avoid the impression that he or she understands the patient better than the parents. This will require careful facilitation skills that probe the parents' understanding and invite them to consider alternative possibilities, without seeming to suggest that they are somehow not being a good advocate for their child.

The cheat sheet is as follows:

1. *Case 16:* The "Ethical Analysis" provided with the case covers several key points. Ethically, the consultant will want Jessica's voice to be heard and help drive the treatment decision making toward palliation. Nevertheless, it is important that the consultant avoid a situation where they and the doctor seem to be ganging up on the patient's mother and thereby hardening her in her position. Asking questions and listening will be helpful, along with gentle nudges that help the patient's mother to consider the goal of palliation—for example, "Have you thought about how a focus on comfort care would differ from what Jessica is currently experiencing?" In cases such as this one, where trust with the physician is in question, offering proactive options such as a second opinion can help build trust with the family.

2. *Case 17:* One question facing an ethics consultant in such a case is, simply, "For whom is one consulting"? That is, you would probably be asked by the administration whether there was any reason they should not compel treatment. As the outcome showed, the danger is the rupture of the provider–family relationship, which could have long-term implications. You will need to decide whether talking with the patient's parents will help you understand the potential for such a rupture, and how that should be weighed against the patient's immediate medical interests. Your goal in a conversation with the parents might be to build the relationship by allowing them to express their opinion and helping them understand the choice the health system was

facing. Such candor might build a sturdier relationship, even after compelling treatment (Pinkus, Smentanka, and Kottkamp 2008, 59–65).

3. *Case 18:* The most difficult part of such cases is often to determine what the options for the patient might be. In the absence of realistic discharge alternatives, facilitating ethical decision making is near impossible. As a result, an ethics consultant will sometimes need to work closely with those who do discharge planning, such as the social worker or case manager for this unit. Finding options, such as a nursing home or rehabilitation facility, can make a good outcome possible.

4. *Case 19:* A case such as this can require that an ethics consultant help all parties, especially the members of the health care team, to analyze the concept of the best interest of a child. This has many elements, including the integrity of the family, in addition to physical concerns, such as not being dropped. In analyzing such a concept, the ethics consultant can help the team to consider whether many of the concerns are as threatening as they seem, or whether we are holding this family to a higher standard than most. Similarly, we can help them to understand that the best interest of the child does not mean the absolute best situation—for example, babies are not reassigned to richer or better-educated parents to maximize their interests. The safety of the child is paramount, rather than an ideal setting. Such an analysis can be helpful in redirecting the conversation toward finding additional home supports for the family.

5. *Case 20:* This is an odd case, in that the patient is not actually a minor chronologically. However, like many patients who have been ill since they were very young, this patient has not developed the independence that is typical of adulthood. An ethics consultant can help gently clarify certain concepts, such as the fact that the patient has the decision-

making capacity and legal rights to make his own decisions. But because the patient's identity and autonomy are seemingly intertwined with those of his parents, a consultant in this kind of case usually must work toward a facilitated consensus. Pitting the wishes of the parents against those of the patient will not likely result in effective decision making by the patient.

6. *Case 21:* This case seems unusual because it is in the rehabilitation setting and involves treatments taking place over a long term. As with many cases, an ethics consultant does well to keep the concepts of goals and treatments front and center. The treating team and the parent had to come to some agreement on what goals can be currently addressed with what therapies. And they needed to agree on the possibilities for reevaluating potential goals and treatments in the future. Keys to the agreed-on resolution were listening to the concerns of the parents, reframing the discussion, and providing acceptable options for all parties.

Conceptual Framework

The ethical framework for making medical decisions that involve pediatric patients takes different starting points than cases involving adults. Of course, pediatric patients are not a uniform population, so decision making may involve various processes, depending on age and capacity—for example, contrast the patients in case 19 (a newborn baby) and case 20 (nearly an adult). In fact, they are a diverse population, and the problems that arise when dealing with newborns and other patients who are so young that they clearly have no capacity to make decisions are very different from the problems of adolescents who have some capacity.

Three issues are worth exploring because they form the background questions and assumptions to most decision making for and with patients who are minors:

1. What does it mean to say that decisions for minors should be made in their best interests?
2. What is the role of the family in such a schema of decision making?
3. Can a minor ever make their own health care decisions?

**Best Interests in Their Purest Form: Experiential
versus Future-Oriented Interests**

The framework for decision making for adult patients relies on the wishes of the patient. This is not possible in the case of children, because they are presumed to lack the capacity to make decisions for themselves. Typically, parents make decisions for their children according to a "best interests" standard. (You will see the word "interest" in both the singular and plural in the literature. The singular version probably refers to a particular outcome of deliberation; i.e., when all is said and done, this particular course of action is the best one and is considered to be in the main interest of the child. But, children, like all of us, have a variety of interests. Thus, many use the plural version, in that it admits that the deliberators are probably seeking the choice that accords with more of the child's interests rather than fewer.) That is, they take into account what is in the child's interests and make decisions accordingly. Children typically have two kinds of interests:

1. Present, experiential interests. These are interests in avoiding pain and suffering, feeling pleasure and comfort, and so on.
2. Future-oriented interests. These are the child's interests in having a future that has opportunities and possibilities for self-fulfillment, among which they may choose (the child's right to an "open future").

It is not always clear which kind of interests we are talking about when we say that a decision should be in the child's best interests. The future-oriented interests are more typically what we associate with specifically being persons, as has been discussed previously. As a result, future-oriented interests are usually the ones that receive primacy. For example, we have few qualms about putting a child

— 155 —

through the immediate pain of a vaccination to safeguard his or her future. We usually argue that it is the child's inability to appreciate these future-oriented interests that make parents the appropriate decision makers.

Most difficulties arise when the patient's forward-looking interests are likely to be truncated. Infants who are severely physically or cognitively impaired may be unlikely to develop the capacities for life plans and other activities that are considered normal for most persons. If the level of impairment is very severe, the patient may have only experiential interests. Judging what level of treatment is in such a baby's best experiential interests is not a simple calculation. There are at least two slightly different estimates of these interests:

1. Life extension outweighs almost everything else: This approach hypothesizes that if we are judging only according to the baby's best experiential interests, we will seldom terminate life-prolonging treatment. There might be exceptions, such as patients who suffer from Lesh-Nyhan syndrome and Tay Sachs disease, who may have pain and suffering that cannot be sufficiently controlled, with the result that continued existence may be more of a burden than a benefit to the child. But it is generally hard to find examples of illnesses in which nonexistence is actually better than existence for the patient (Strong 1984).

2. Pain, suffering, and other burdens are often the most salient and decisive factors; conversely, others claim that even on an experiential model of best interests, we must not underestimate the suffering caused by repeated procedures, iatrogenic illnesses, and other difficulties associated with many ongoing infirmities. Although a specific condition might not be associated with constant pain, life in institutional

environments is stressful, difficult, and generally invasive. If one cannot understand why the discomforts associated with treatments are being inflicted, the discomforts and indignities may feel assaultive and cruel, and thereby be highly burdensome. This approach argues that treatment may be forgone in order to relieve the patient of the considerable burdens these treatments and hospitalizations inflict. Such an argument in favor of declining treatment is simply a version of the doctrine of double-effect thinking (Buchanan and Brock 1990, 215–66).

Who Calculates Best Interests? The Role of the Family

Traditionally, neonatal units have been known to have an environment of paternalism that is second to none. Contrary to this clinical cultural norm, there seems to be a societal consensus that parents should ultimately determine what is in their child's best interests, within certain limits (the Baby Doe cases helped us to ascertain what those limits might be). The reason behind this belief is not exactly clear: Several candidates are:

1. Parents love their children. Parents generally have the child's interests at heart. Best interest is not a completely objective determination. Therefore, we should let those who care most about the child make such a determination, because they are likely to do it best.
2. Their decisions are as good as any. Many decisions involving newborns with severe impairments or congenital anomalies have a high degree of uncertainty. Therefore, there is no single right answer, and the judgment should rest with those who will live with the outcomes.

3. Parents must live with the consequences. In fact, what is in the child's best interest will depend, in part, on what the parents are willing or have the capacity to do for the child.

4. Parents and other family members also have interests and rights. Society cannot demand that these persons sacrifice all opportunities—including opportunities for their other children, perhaps their marriages, and other basic life projects—to the care of one severely debilitated family member. For instance, parents may have several children, and it is important that all the children have some parental support. This may sound harsh in a culture that places a premium on the individual. It may sound less harsh to some from more communally oriented cultures.

5. Society has an interest in strong family units. Allowing families to be the ultimate arbiter of decisions strengthens them.

What is clear from these considerations is that though we must make medical decisions with the interests of the minor patient as the most important factor, the interests of the child and the family unit are intertwined and, at times, inseparable. Thus, clinical ethics consultants and health care professionals should avoid pitting the interests of patient and family against each other whenever possible. The more the members of the family unit thrive and maintain their integrity, the better they are able to support the patient.

In general, violating the integrity of the family to provide treatment to a minor patient over parental objections is best justified when the intervention is likely to be curative, is easily administered, and has minimal burdens. The less clear the benefits of the treatment, the more reluctant one should be to override the decision-making prerogative of families.

Children and Decision-Making Capacity: Can Children Ever Make Their Own Health Care Decisions?

The question of whether children ever make their own health care decisions has several dimensions:

1. Presumption of incompetence: Children are usually assumed to lack the cognitive or evaluative mechanisms necessary for good medical decision making. This is the reverse of the situation regarding adults. With adults, we initially presume that they possess decision-making capacity.

2. Normally, we work with a model that requires parental consent and the patient's assent. The parent looks after the child's best interests and safeguards their future autonomy; the child's dignity is respected with the provision of information and by procuring the assent of the child when possible.

3. Decision-making capacity is not an all-or-nothing affair. As a general rule of thumb, the older the child, the more likely they are to have more of the elements of capacity. Of course, individual cases vary.

4. Children who wish to participate in decision making may have their capacity evaluated. In general, we are looking for the same abilities to understand information, to apply a relatively stable set of values to their choices, and to appreciate the consequences of their decisions.

5. The statuses of mature minor and emancipated minor are available in many states to allow certain minors to exercise their autonomy and self-determination. Typically, a child is declared a mature minor by the courts for the purposes of making a single health care decision—for example, declining a round of chemotherapy that her parents want her to have—when the patient can demonstrate the usual requisites for

being judged competent. A child is usually declared to be an emancipated minor by satisfying certain criteria in the state's statute—for example, living on his or her own and financial self-sufficiency. Emancipated minors possess the full decision-making rights of adults with regard to their health care decisions.

In clinical practice, problems are seldom of the variety where the child insists on making a decision and no one will let him or her do so. More commonly, we see parents who are used to protecting their child not soliciting opinions from the patient and not acknowledging that their child's wishes may be developing contrary to their own. In other words, chronic illness can make a person rather passive and prevent an adolescent from forming the normal independence and autonomy that most show. Then, the question becomes how far health care providers should go in being the "patient's advocate."

Case 20 shows an adult man who has essentially been kept in the child's role when it comes to decision making about his health care. Because he has had a long-term chronic illness since he was so young, his parents never really recognized that their role should evolve away from being so "parental"—that is, paternalistic. This young man actually did live away from his parents for a time, and was once married. However, he remained their sick child in their minds, and they never came to afford him autonomy in their relationship. Thus, when he moved home to be cared for, old patterns of decision making emerged.

This case is instructive. By analogy, we can imagine how hard it must be for, say, a sixteen-year-old patient with cystic fibrosis who has been cared for all his life at home. His parents became used to making medical decisions for him for many years, and they may never have come to include their son in decision making, despite the fact that his cognitive and affective abilities have developed to warrant it. The concept of "assent" is important, given these states of quasi-capacity. This concept requires that the patient be given information from the earliest possible age, even though he has no substantive role in decision making. It is almost as if the patient is in training for giving fully informed consent when he has developed the capabilities.

Of course, clinical practice is a varied place, and one may come across unusual variations of these scenarios over time. However, using the conceptual framework of best interests, we are prepared to analyze and address such variations. For instance, the case of Cassandra C received much media attention (Cassandra C. 2015). She presented as a seventeen-year-old patient who wished to refuse highly beneficial treatment (which was likely to be curative) for Hodgkin's lymphoma and be supported in dying. It was unusual because her mother also supported her in this contention. Despite these permutations, the issues of best interest, family integrity, and the increasing decision-making capacity of the patient are all in evidence and are available for analysis.

References and Further Reading

Buchanan, Allen, and Dan W. Brock. 1990. *Deciding for Others: The Ethics of Surrogate Decision Making*. New York: Cambridge University Press.

Cassandra C. 2015. "This Is My Life and My Body." *Hartford Courant*, January 8. www.courant.com/opinion/op-ed/hc-op-cassandra-my-body-my-life-0109-20150108-story.html.

Lee, K. Jane, Kelly Tieves, and Mathew Scanlon. 2010. "Alterations in End-of-Life Support in the Pediatric Intensive Care Unit." *Pediatrics*. 126, no. 4: e859–e864.

Luce, John M. 2010. "A History of Resolving Conflicts over End-of-Life Care in Intensive Care Units in the United States." *Critical Care Medicine* 38: 1623–29.

McCabe, Megan, Elizabeth A. Hunt, and Janet R. Serwint. 2008. "Pediatric Residents' Clinical and Educational Experiences with End-of-Life Care." *Pediatrics* 121, no. 4: 731–37.

Pinkus, Rosa Lynn, Stella L. Smentanka, and Nathan A. Kottkamp. 2008. "Suzie's Voice." In *Complex Ethics Consultations: Cases That Haunt Us*, edited by P. Ford and D. Dudzinski. New York: Cambridge University Press.

Placencia, Frank X., and Laurence B. McCullough. 2011. "The History of Ethical Decision Making in Neonatal Intensive Care." *Journal of Intensive Care Medicine* 26: 368–84.

Strong, Carson. 1984. "The Neonatologist's Duty to Patient and Parents." *Hastings Center Report* 14, no. 4: 10–16.

SECTION IV

ORGANIZATIONAL ETHICS

Case 22:
"If We Do This, They'll All Come Here"
A Kidney Transplant for
an Undocumented Immigrant?

SKILL BUILDER CASE: This case is designed for building clinical ethics consultation skills through simulation. Visit the ACES website for a video enacting this consultation and skills assessment materials at LUC.edu/ethicsconsult/.

Key Terms: *Access to Care, Charity Care, Health Care Disparities, Mission Leadership, Kidney Transplantation, Undocumented Immigrants*

Narrative

The patient, Mr. D, is a fifty-six-year-old man who suffers from end-stage renal disease. He has a variety of health issues, including diabetes. Fortunately, his diabetes has been well managed through diet, lifestyle adjustments, and insulin injections. He has been receiving dialysis at a dialysis center affiliated with your health system for about four years. When his kidney failure began, he would present at your Emergency Department, and he would receive "emergency dialysis," which was covered by the state's Medicaid program. However, after a couple of months, your institution decided to ask him to come to the dialysis center twice a week for dialysis and to absorb the cost of this care as part of your facility's charity care budget. This approach seemed prudent because regularly scheduled dialysis should result in a significantly better quality of life and related health outcomes.

Mr. D. is a good candidate for a kidney transplant, given that his health problems are relatively well controlled. If he were a citizen of the United States, he would likely be placed on the waiting list by your health system's transplant program. The dialysis of a citizen would be covered by Medicare, which would pay for the transplantation surgery and several years of the needed posttransplant immunosuppressive medications. The state's expanded Medicaid coverage would assist a citizen in his situation to obtain their medication after the Medicare benefits ran out. Unfortunately, a person with an unauthorized immigration status is ineligible for these benefits.

In recent months, Mr. D's pastor has taken up his cause. Pastor Valdez leads a Pentecostal congregation that is increasingly becoming known for its activism on behalf of undocumented immigrants. He has begun doing social media activism to "call out" the transplant programs in the area, and he has recently escalated his activities. He and members of the congregation picketed outside a neighboring hospital requesting a meeting with the chief executive officer (CEO) about their transplant program. His activism is garnering a modest amount of media coverage, and he is likely to do similar events at other hospitals, potentially including yours. Several members of the congregation have said on social media and in public that they would be willing to give Mr. D one of their kidneys (but none have yet gone through the matching process at a transplant program).

As the director of the ethics consultation service, you are contacted to attend a meeting that is being organized by your CEO to discuss this case. It is not clear exactly what question or questions will form the focus of the meeting.

Perspectives for Role Players

Dr. Fitzpatrick [played by a physician or actor]:

- Dr. Fitzpatrick is the chief medical officer of the health system.
- You believe patients should generally get the appropriate care for their condition.
- You see transplantation as superior to indefinite dialysis for Mr. D.
- You recognize that many patients placed on a waiting list never actually receive a kidney.
- You think it is hard to gauge how many potential living donors from Mr. D's congregation would go through the matching and donation process. So the likelihood of having a living donor available is not entirely clear.
- You are not sure what criteria should govern which undocumented immigrants you will do transplants for and which you will not.
- The fact that Mr. D has been a patient in this health system for an extended period elicits some sympathy from you. After all, he is "our patient," and the health system has been absorbing his dialysis costs.
- You are rather sure that a surgeon or two on staff would donate their time for the surgery. The main challenge will be paying for the immunosuppressive medications on an ongoing basis.

Vik Singh [played by an actor]:

- Mr. Singh is the chief financial officer of the hospital.
- You consistently refer to undocumented immigrants as "those people" or "illegals."

- Your main concern is payer mix. You see no advantage to offering a free service to anyone, even though you accept that some emergency service must be offered by law.
- You try not to seem offensive, because you understand that some of the others in the room like to talk about "mission" with regard to uncompensated care and you need to not seem hostile to such talk.

Dr. P. Taylor [played by an actor]:

- P. Taylor is the CEO of the health system.
- You are very proud of the way that the health system carries out its charity care mission.
- Currently, you see immigrant populations as a fiscal challenge to the health system. But in the health system's future, these people and their children are likely to become the most important patient population. So you work hard on establishing good relations with this community.
- You want a creative solution that enables the health system to do some cases of this type but does not attract so many similar cases as to deluge the system.
- You are open to the hospital's charity care fund providing an ongoing contribution to the purchase of immunosuppressants if other contributors—for example, the community and the pharmaceutical companies—will share some responsibility.

Ethics Consultant [played by you]:

- You are concerned about the plight of this patient and other undocumented patients who seem unfairly excluded from the benefits of transplantation. However, you are realistic and realize that charity care is a limited resource.

- You understand that in your market, your health system cannot become the lone willing provider of such services. To take on such a role would place your health system at a large competitive fiscal disadvantage: "No margin, no mission."
- You have two goals for the meeting: (1) to be sure that undocumented immigrants are discussed with respect for their situation and that biases (e.g., referring to them as "illegals") do not color any decision regarding the potential use of charity care funds and (2) to get the health system to make a commitment of some magnitude to assist this patient population regarding transplantation and begin to develop appropriate supporting criteria. Although the hospital cannot "do everything," you believe that it can make a commitment to doing some level of this kind of work.
- It is not clear by what criteria the health system might choose to provide a transplant and follow-up care to a particular undocumented immigrant patient.

Ethical Analysis

This kind of case has been increasingly common in health care systems in the United States (Lee 2015). Many researchers estimate that the United States has between 10 and 12 million people with an undocumented immigration status. The US Congress has failed to enact any kind of immigration reform that would make possible the adjustment of the immigration status of these members of the community. As long as they remain undocumented (and in the current legal system, there is no path to correct this situation for most undocumented immigrants), they are ineligible for any government benefits, such as access to Medicare or Medicaid. Thus, the health care financing systems that usually support dialysis and transplantation fail the health care facility in these instances.

There are two attitudes and assumptions that an ethicist must call into question in this kind of discussion. The first is simple dismissal of such a case, with an assertion that "We'd like to help, but we simply can't afford to do so." Although resources are limited, and a health system may not be able to meet the need for all services if it has a high prevalence of uninsured, undocumented patients in its census area, some resources must undoubtedly be devoted to such a population. The legal obligations specified by the Emergency Medical Treatment and Labor Act to treat patients who present for emergency care mean that health systems must treat a patient who presents in kidney failure until he is stabilized. As a result, the case presented can be seen as a stage in a larger deliberation about how best—perhaps, how most efficiently—to discharge such obligations. This patient is probably receiving dialysis on a regular schedule under the health system's charity care policy, because this is clearly better for the patient's health than having the patient repeatedly present in extremis in the emergency room and then dialyzing him. Both approaches require the use of resources, and the former one constitutes much better health care.

Second, the ethicist must help to facilitate a discussion that is appropriately respectful of this patient, and similarly situated patients, as patients presenting from the community that the health system serves (Wasson and Cook 2014). Health care professionals, as professionals, do not treat some patients as worthy of their respect and others as not. When such patients present, the ethical obligations of the providers and the system are the same as for any other patient. Some prefacing of the discussion with terminological clarifications would be an important starting point. Thus, the ethicist could stipulate that any reference to the patient's immigration status be given as "undocumented" rather than "illegal." Relatedly, though such a case conference takes place away from the clinic floor, clinicians feel a professional obligation to treat like patients alike, regardless of their insurance status. Thus, an inability to facilitate an equitable solution should be seen as potentially undermining a clinical ethos that the institution strives to foster. Therefore, to whatever extent possible, this patient should be seen simply as a patient, and the goal should be to provide the same standard of care that any other patient would receive (Kuczewski 2017).

The reality is that charity care resources are limited, and thus criteria for their responsible stewardship must be developed. In the clinical case on which this role play is based, the community organizations supporting this patient's public campaign for a transplant were challenged to fund-raise for the immunosuppressive medications that the patient would need for the rest of his life. They raised enough money to provide medication for several years. The surgeon and consulting physicians donated their services. The health system agreed to seek donated and discounted medications from the pharmaceutical company—and, in addition, to fill any gaps, so the patient would receive immunosuppressive medications indefinitely, which likely means the rest of his life. The health system cannot take on many similar indefinite obligations. Thus, criteria are being considered that might limit the number of such obligations; for example, a patient would need to be a dialysis patient at the facility for a defined number of years before being considered for a transplant. In short, a creative solution was found that enabled each party to honor its values without unrealistically jeopardizing its resources. That is an ideal outcome.

Case 23:
"But She's *Our* Patient"
Margin and Medical Mission

Key Terms: *Medical Mission, Organizational Ethics, Uncompensated Care*

Narrative

Fred Granholm, MD, is the CEO of a large health system, Oak Valley–Mercy Health. One morning, he receives a call from Dr. Frank Clavell, a young, up-and-coming cardiovascular surgeon in this health system. He handles a reasonable number of cases in your institution, but he also works at one or two other hospitals. Because Dr. Clavell's practice will continue to grow significantly, Dr. Granholm, as CEO, is very interested in having him bring all his cases to Oak Valley–Mercy Health.

Dr. Clavell's request is a complicated one. While on a recent mission trip to a rural area of Colombia, he encountered a patient with a heart problem that he says is a septal defect—or at least that is what he believes, given the limited diagnostic tools available to him in that environment. This patient is a twenty-seven-year-old mother of two children who is 23 weeks pregnant. He has grave concerns that given what he could assess about her, she might not survive another delivery. He would like to fly her up to Oak Valley–

Mercy Health and perform a septal defect repair on her. If she goes into early labor or if, in consultation with the high-risk obstetrics team, she should need a C-section, then she would also deliver her baby at Oak Valley–Mercy Health. Then the baby could be cared for in the neonatal intensive care unit until he or she was strong enough to return to Colombia with the mother.

Dr. Clavell is willing to perform this surgery gratis, as is one of his anesthesia colleagues. He wants the hospital to also provide free care.

The Language and Issues of the Case

As with many organizational ethics issues, we do not necessarily have a readily developed terminology or language for this case. Although there is a small but developing literature on ethical issues in medical mission trips, there is not much relevant literature regarding the ethics of this kind of negotiation between the CEO and Dr. Clavell. Nevertheless, we know that this case raises questions of how the health system defines and circumscribes its mission:

1. Is it ethical for Dr. Granholm to use this situation to secure a more exclusive contractual relationship for the health system with Dr. Clavell?
2. How should a health care system balance its duty to local underserved populations with international or national service work? Are there reasons to do local charity work exclusively? Or are there reasons to do some work beyond one's local or regional catchment area?
3. Is it ever a moral duty to bring a patient from another country to your facility for treatment? What kind of criteria might make doing so appropriate?

Section IV

Perspectives and Key Points of View

Dr. Fred Granholm (CEO of Oak Valley–Mercy Health): He is interested in making Dr. Clavell happy and sees this particular request as
doable from a business standpoint. That is, even if things do not go
well, the total expenses incurred by the health system could be
absorbed and would be a reasonable price to pay if it meant gaining
Dr. Clavell's exclusive loyalty. Dr. Granholm sees nothing wrong in
bonding with a clinician over the hospital's charitable mission. But
he also has two main concerns. First, he is concerned that if he simply accepts this patient without directly negotiating for more of Dr.
Clavell's volumes, he will set a bad precedent and end up being
ineffectual in his ultimate goal. It is hard to negotiate with a physician in Colombia without seeming crass. And second, if he accepts
this patient, he would hope to keep it quiet. Local leaders could
become angry at the exorbitant use of uncompensated care for
someone from another country while resources are strained for local
community health programs.

    Dr. Frank Clavell: He thinks this case is a no-brainer for Dr. Gran-
holm. After all, the medical mission trip is being sponsored by the
health system. Oak Valley–Mercy Health is very proud of its service,
and this is "their patient." Furthermore, this will make a great story
and garner much favorable media attention. Dr. Clavell sees this
case as a rare opportunity to do a lot of good very easily and live up
to the mission that Dr. Granholm touts passionately.

    Ethics Consultant: The ethics consultant dislikes having to be the
naysayer in these kinds of cases, but generally he does not think
well of such proposals. Although they sometimes can go well and
be good for morale at the hospital, they can easily go poorly, owing
to a misdiagnosis in the field. And once the patient has been removed
from her home environment, she will not have any familial social
support when bad news or a poor outcome ensues. As a result, the
consultant favors devoting resources to assisting people in their

home environments and thus developing a health care network at the point of service. The ethics consultant is less concerned about the overall resource allocation issue, because it is difficult to say when too much is being spent in one area or another from an ethical standpoint.

What Actually Happened

Dr. Granholm agreed to the plan to bring the patient to Oak Valley–Mercy Health. He did not directly raise a quid pro quo with Dr. Clavell but hoped to soon have a mission-focused conversation about Dr. Clavell's future as a leader in the system. The patient's examination and work-up at Oak Valley–Mercy Health ruled out a septal defect, and a precise diagnosis was difficult. The patient was found to be in partial heart failure, which was treated with medication. Idiopathic cardiomyopathy was the diagnosis on which Dr. Clavell settled. The high-risk obstetrics team wished for the patient to continue gestation as long as possible. The patient stayed on a general medicine floor for a full month, until a C-section delivery was scheduled and completed. The baby was born and was in good health. Both the baby and the mother were returned to Colombia two weeks after the baby's birth. The mother died suddenly at home approximately one year later. The child continues to thrive.

Case 24:
Charity Care—
What Are the Criteria?

Key Terms: *Charity Care, Discharge Planning*

Narrative

Ms. C is a forty-seven-year-old woman who is a ventilator dependent quadriplegic, with multiple medical problems, including diabetes. A home care agency that is affiliated with a large Catholic
nonprofit health system has cared for her for several years. She was
initially treated at the affiliated hospital following an accident, and
her family physician is part of the system's physician network.

Ms. C receives daily in-home services from a registered nurse
and an aide—including for control of her diabetes, tracheostomy
care, a bowel program, physical therapy, bathing, and so on. A respiratory therapist also visits on occasion to maintain the ventilator in
good order.

Ms. C has always had commercial insurance with good home
care coverage. This insurance has been provided through her
spouse's employer, which has changed insurance carriers several
times in recent years; but fortunately, coverage has remained fairly
good. This past year, the employer chose a new insurance carrier

and coverage again changed, but within three months the client had hit the annual cap on her home care benefits for the year.

The patient is not eligible for Medicare due to not being home-bound. (She gets out with her motorized wheelchair.) Medicaid benefits were investigated, and Medicaid approved home care benefits as medically necessary, in amounts of service similar to what she has been receiving. However, Medicaid has a maximum reimbursement that equals the amount they pay to maintain a person in a long-term care facility. In other words, Medicaid will not pay more to keep someone at home than they would to keep them in a nursing home, currently costing nearly $3,000 per month.

The amount Medicaid will pay is substantially less than the agency cost of placing the care providers in the home. Care for this client would create an annual loss of approximately $12,000. Such a sum is a considerable amount of write-off, and it has the possibility to increase soon (e.g., Medicaid has asked the agency to investigate reducing the services provided). The client wants this care provided as charity and states, "You've made plenty of money off me." The client meets the health system's basic charity care guidelines.

Should the agency use charity care dollars to fund this client's decision to stay home when the client does have another option—that is, long-term care—and those charity dollars could be used for home care patients who do not have that option? In addition, the home care agency has been operating in the red this past year due to recent changes in home care reimbursement. These changes have caused the health system to schedule a process of review and discernment to determine what its commitment to providing home care services should be.

The Language and Issues of the Case

This case involves the balancing of "margin and mission" that is common in nonprofit health care and is, perhaps, made more explicitly thematic in faith-based institutions. Charity care has generally been discussed in terms of services provided by a hospital to patients through the Emergency Department or who are admitted to in-patient services through the Emergency Department. Because large health systems now involve a larger array of kinds of care that extend further into the community, cases such as this one raise questions about the scope and reach of a local health care system's charity commitment:

1. Given that the need for in-home services is high but coverage for such services is often limited, how can one describe criteria that enable the health system to carry out its mission but do not result in an unrealistic financial burden for the system?
2. What aspects of Ms. C's case make her a good candidate for charity care? What factors mitigate against it?
3. Is it ethically defensible for a health system to choose to provide charity care for some parts of its system (for example, acute services) but not others (for example, home care)? How could one ethically justify such a policy? What ethical considerations argue against a policy of this type?

Perspectives and Key Points of View

Vice president for mission and ethics: The role of vice president for mission, which is common in large Catholic health systems, is filled by a person who seeks to be sure that the institution's values and mission are integrated into all its major policies and decisions. This vice president felt that there was a good case for providing ongoing home care to Ms. C. After all, she was a longtime patient of the health system, and her evolving insurance coverage situation was not her doing. Furthermore, there was a payer—that is, Medicaid—although this payer underfunds the needed care. Nevertheless, the case for absorbing some loss and working over time to minimize that loss was far better than if there were no payer and only loss to be incurred. The health system might learn more about efficiency and best practices by working toward minimizing that loss. This vice president also found it hard to know how to make the trade-off between this patient's care and devoting those resources to others in need of charity care. But the fact that Medicaid would cover a significant part of the cost meant that denying this patient further services would not provide enough savings to assist a patient who had no insurance. Thus, there is a kind of efficacy rationale for this investment by the hospital.

Chief financial officer: The chief financial officer is always interested in seeing that the institution's charity care policy is implemented in a relatively consistent and defensible way. He is motivated to be sure that long-term charity care commitments not become so numerous that they crowd out immediate acute needs in the future. Thus, he could be open to this case as the patient meets the general charity care criteria. He needs an analysis that suggests that this patient's profile and the criteria she meets are not likely to fit many other patients. If this is the case, then his main concerns have been allayed.

What Actually Happened

After significant deliberation, the health system decided that it would continue to provide in-home services to Ms. C and accept the Medicaid payment. It would use charity care funds to offset whatever losses were incurred. It based this conclusion on its long-term relationship with the patient and its desire to maintain the level of services and living arrangement with which the patient thrived. The health system also innovated in a number of ways by working with close family members to train them to provide some of the patient's support on an intermittent basis and reduce costs. The patient died after approximately four years under this arrangement.

Case 25:
"What's the Use?"
Capacity, Addiction, and Fairness

⚜
Key Terms: *Substance Use Disorder, Nonadherence*
⚜

Narrative

A cardiac surgeon, Dr. Thomas, requested an ethics consultation regarding a twenty-seven-year-old woman, Ms. N, who needs a repeat surgery for endocarditis—that is, an infected heart valve. The patient is known to the requesting physician. He treated her for this condition two years ago by placing a prosthetic heart valve. Dr. Thomas is seeking an ethics consultation to advise him whether he should perform the surgery again, because the patient repeatedly infects herself through intravenous (IV) drug use. The physician states that "repeatedly treating this patient for endocarditis and related complications is a waste of health care resources and amounts to futile care because the patient will not stop abusing drugs." The patient has had three previous admissions for endocarditis, the last of which involved Dr. Thomas performing the replacement of the infected heart valve.

The first two times the patient was admitted, she was treated with IV drug therapy, and Dr. Thomas has considered focusing on this approach again. However, the patient has consistently resisted remaining in the hospital to complete long-term IV antibiotic therapy, and she likens it to imprisonment. During one of her previous visits, she requested to be discharged to her mother's home with home health services to complete her IV therapy, but the clinical team refused to facilitate that discharge plan for fear that she might use her IV access to inject illegal drugs. The patient left the hospital against medical advice one time after completing four of the prescribed six weeks of IV antibiotics.

The Language and Issues of the Case

Such a case is often discussed under the headings of noncompliance, nonadherence, and rationing care based on fiscal scarcity (i.e., costs). Of course, the noncompliance or nonadherence is owing to addiction, a substance use disorder. IV drug users and the treatment of their infections is beginning to generate a small ethical literature of its own, largely owing to the increased frequency of this kind of dilemma (see also case 7). Some questions on which an ethics consultation might focus include:

1. What is the relative efficacy of valve replacement versus not replacing it? That is, though it might seem ineffective to replace it if the patient continues to use IV drugs, what would be the expected outcome of replacing it versus not doing so? Are there some benefits even if she continues to use illegal substances?
2. Are there any other analogous situations in which physicians deny a nonadherent patient needed therapy for reasons of fiscal scarcity? Or would this be an anomalous situation?
3. What resources are available for supporting any attempt the patient may be willing to make to stop using illegal substances?

Case 25: What's the Use?

Perspectives and Key Points of View

Dr. Thomas (cardiac surgeon): This surgeon would like to effectively treat the patient. However, he believes that surgery will be effective for a limited time and that the patient will again infect the valve through her IV drug use. He thinks that he is in some way enabling her substance use disorder by continually replacing the valve. It is difficult for him to articulate exactly how he comes to this conclusion. But it seems that by doing these valve replacements, he is somehow reassuring the patient that he can effectively treat her illness. Her continued drug use will, however, likely eventually result in an infection that will take her life. He is very frustrated.

Ms. N (the patient): Ms. N cannot believe that this situation keeps happening to her. After all, she is young, and though many people's drug habits are far worse than hers, they do not keep ending up in the hospital. Also, few things make her want "to use" more than being cooped up in the hospital. She would really like to cut down on her drug use, so she has tried some of the typical approaches to recovery, such as attending a few Narcotics Anonymous meetings. But they have not led to long-term recovery. She might be interested in trying a different approach. She alternates between being terrified of dying and thinking it might be for the best.

Ethics Consultant: The ethics consultant's analysis is that denying the patient surgery will be difficult to justify ethically. Failure to make lifestyle changes that prevent recurrent illness is seldom seen as a reason to deny treatment, unless it involves use of a scarce commodity, such as a solid organ for transplantation. In cases of commodity scarcity, the commodity—that is, the organ—would be denied another patient by providing it to the noncompliant patient. The consultant is also concerned that the patient be given a realistic opportunity for treatment of her substance use disorder—that is, she will be told that she needs to stop using drugs. However, realistic treatment options for such a patient are seldom provided or available.

What Actually Happened

A psychiatry consultation was requested. Although the patient remained clearly ambivalent about treatment, she agreed to explore options. With the help of a social worker, the patient was able to find an in-patient rehabilitation program that agreed to take her once her endocarditis had been successfully treated. Dr. Thomas scheduled and performed the valve replacement. The hospital agreed to keep the patient in the hospital for a week longer than usual so she would be strong enough to go to the in-patient rehabilitation center immediately after discharge. During that week, she received visits from alumnae of a rehabilitation program and other members of Narcotics Anonymous. The patient was successful in her attempts to stay free of IV drug use for approximately two years, at which time she again began injecting IV drugs. She presented soon thereafter at the hospital with chills and a fever. She was diagnosed as again having endocarditis.

Case 26:
A Teaching Hospital's
Transfer Policy—
Who Is Responsible for This Patient?

Key Terms: *Transfer Policy, Head Trauma, Physician–Patient Relationships, Inter-Hospital Relationships, Referral Relationships, Standard of Care*

Narrative

Dr. Stansfield, the chief medical officer at the main hospital of Johnson University Health System (JUHS), receives a text page at about 7 pm from one of the senior neurosurgeons, Dr. Rocca. When Dr. Stansfield phones Dr. Rocca, he learns that Dr. Rocca, the neurosurgeon on call this evening, is upset about a call his resident just received. The resident relayed to him that a local community hospital emergency room (ER) is requesting a transfer for a patient who seems to have an intracranial hemorrhage and has asked Dr. Rocca to call the ER physician about the potential transfer.

When Dr. Rocca called the physician at the community hospital's ER, Dr. Sheila Reed, the physician described a patient who has been in their ER for four hours awaiting the neurosurgeon from their medical staff. Dr. Rocca is familiar with this particular private practice neurosurgeon and believes that he knows quite a bit about him—for example, he is on staff at four hospitals, and, like many neurosurgeons, he is not at all thrilled about doing trauma work because it has a high malpractice risk and does not pay comparatively well. But rotating through trauma call is entailed by his practice group's contract with the four hospitals. Dr. Reed is concerned that the patient is decompensating and is anxious to transfer that patient out of her busy ER. She does not know for certain, but she said something about believing the patient waited a long time to come to the hospital because she is uninsured. English is not the patient's primary language, and Dr. Reed is not certain she got the whole story accurately.

Dr. Rocca is upset because this is about the fourth call that he and his partners have received from that hospital in the past three weeks where the neurosurgeons seem to never be available for this type of head trauma. Dr. Rocca's opinion is that this patient will not likely need surgical intervention but will be in the hospital for several days for observation, initially in an intensive care unit. Dr. Rocca thinks that such observation could probably be done in the community hospital, by neurology or neurosurgery.

The Language and Issues of the Case

The difficulty in finding a framework with which to analyze this case is that obligations to patients generally derive from physician–patient relationships. There are few developed frameworks for obligations to persons with whom a physician or a hospital has not yet entered into a relationship. Nevertheless, the hospital's mission might provide some opportunity for considering potential responsibilities. Questions to consider include:

1. Are there any acceptable alternatives for this patient? Failure to identify one alternative perhaps engages the health system in a prima facie duty to rescue.

2. What is the long-term impact of whatever decision is made? For instance, would allowing this particular patient to receive less than the standard of care solve the problems Dr. Rocca has noted?
3. Who needs to fix the identified problem, and how?

Perspectives and Key Points of View

Dr. Rocca (neurosurgeon at JUHS): He sees it as his duty to receive patients who need the services and expertise that can only be provided by a level one trauma center, such as the one at JUHS. But he is very frustrated by what he sees as outside practices "taking advantage" of his availability by turfing cases to JUHS that could easily be treated at outside hospitals, especially if their medical staff members "did their jobs." He fears that the very liberal transfer policy of your hospital, which essentially accepts all referrals, simply encourages this behavior. He wonders if it is time for Dr. Stansfield to "send a message" that discourages this behavior.

Dr. Reed (ER physician at a local community hospital): Dr. Reed feels very "stuck in the middle." She knows that this patient probably does not need the attention of a neurosurgeon. Nevertheless, she believes that such a judgment would be better made by a neurosurgeon than her. The patient needs to be admitted to a hospital soon, because the ER is definitely not the place for her. But if Dr. Reed admits her to her community hospital and the patient needs the intervention of a neurosurgeon, she worries that she has placed the patient at risk and will likely be sued for negligence. Although she knows that bypassing her hospital's neurosurgeons could cause some blowback, she feels that she needs to secure a higher level of support for this patient very soon.

Dr. Stansfield (chief medical officer at Johnson University Hospital): He is definitely sympathetic to Dr. Rocca's position. The failure of on-call services at outside hospitals to shoulder their appropriate responsibilities definitely places a greater burden on services offered by his medical staff. As chief medical officer, Dr. Stansfield would like to see his neurosurgical staff freed up to practice "at the top of their licenses" rather than spend a lot of call time on cases that do not require their specific expertise. Nevertheless, he has two concerns in this case. The first is simply for the patient. Although the on-call neurosurgeon at the outside hospital may be negligent, Dr. Stansfield also feels that his hospital would be at fault if it actually let a patient be harmed to make an example of the outside hospital's staff. The second concern is that Dr. Stansfield sees the hospital's transfer policy as ultimately helpful to the well-being of the health system. That is, if outside physicians know they will always get an affirmative response, JUHS will be their first choice for referrals. Conversely, if he lets a physician who is in a tough spot like Dr. Reed down, JUHS will not likely receive transfers from her in the future.

What Actually Happened

Dr. Stansfield and Dr. Rocca quickly came to an agreement that they should accept this patient. Dr. Stansfield offered to represent this problem to the next meeting of the CEO's cabinet. At that meeting, the CEO and the chief medical officer decided to seek a telephone conference with their counterparts from the outside community hospital. In that conference, they discussed the need for the coverage at the outside hospital to be more responsive in a timely fashion. Dr. Stansfield and the CEO reassured the outside hospital that they wished to be of help when needed, but that some of these situations seemed to not serve the patients well. Dr. Stansfield pointed out that in this case, the patient would have been at less risk being observed by the neurosurgery service at the outside hospital. After she was transferred to JUHS, she was judged not to need surgery and was released with medication after observation. Thus, she incurred the additional stress and risk of transfer with no additional service or expertise being provided. The CEO and chief medical officer of the outside hospital were in complete agreement, and they planned to address this matter with their neurosurgery group.

Practical Commentary and Tips on Organizational Ethics, with a Cheat Sheet for Dealing with Cases 22 through 26

Health system administrators may seldom make use of clinical ethicists when faced with issues that could directly affect the institution's operating margin. They may simply see such issues as involving policy decisions that are beyond the scope and expertise of a clinical ethicist. And because senior administrators are key stewards of institutional resources, they may fear that ethicists will unrealistically advocate for treatment of particular patients that, if generalized, would be fiscally unsustainable. In some health systems, particularly large Catholic health care systems, there may be a position at the vice president level that is charged with "mission integration." This person is often included in policy deliberations and seeks to ensure that the values associated with the system's religious founders or sponsors are considered when making important choices. Of course, because organizational ethics issues sometimes first present as clinical cases similar to those analyzed in this section, a person who conducts ethics case consultations may first encounter these issues. In such instances, the ethicist may be involved in escalating the case to the attention of administrators at a higher level.

The key to sound ethical analysis—whether by a professional ethicist, a mission leader, or a health system administrator—is to balance the institutional mission to help vulnerable patients with the fiduciary duty to preserve the margin that makes the hospital's functioning possible. "No margin, no mission" has been an oft-repeated truism of nonprofit health care. This is, in essence, a version of the ethicist's dictum, "Ought implies can." Of course, without confidence that the health system is acting on its mission, there is little reason for the ethicist or community to be concerned about the health system's margin.

Although we usually associate being practical with having immediate answers, organizational ethics generally requires working toward a longer-term policy. In each case, one must aim to set a potentially appropriate precedent. Those who are charged with stewardship of resources are usually most concerned that a precedent will be set that is unsustainable from a fiscal viewpoint—that is, it would be unsustainable to treat similar cases similarly in the future. Thus, in each instance, it is important that the solution recommended in the case contain specific criteria explaining why this case should be handled in such a way and that these criteria be reasonably generalizable.

The cheat sheet is as follows:

1. *Case 22:* This case highlights the challenge clearly. That is, the ethicist wants to help the institution consider criteria that might enable a principled way to accept responsibility for providing such care to some patients but not to become overwhelmed by similar cases in virtue of becoming the only known provider for all undocumented patients in need of organ transplantation. For example, seeking criteria that might prioritize some patients and thereby define responsibility—such as significant time as a dialysis

patient in your system—provides a starting point. Similarly, because community pressure is partly forcing this issue, seeking to engage the community to provide a contribution toward the patient's long-term needs is an option. See the "Ethical Analysis" that immediately follows the case for additional considerations.

2. *Case 23:* As with most organizational ethics cases, this one presents as a clinical case, but long-term policy is at issue. An ethics consultant will ultimately want to help transition the institution's medical mission program from one that "parachutes in" to deliver care—and, in this case, airlifts out a patient—to a more sustainable model. Increasingly, medical missions are based on partnerships with local providers and offer a supportive, educational role to enhance the capabilities of and resources available to local caregivers. Thus, it will be important not to alienate the enthusiasm of Dr. Clavell for his mission efforts but to begin a relationship in which you work toward a more effective approach to realizing this mission (Stone and Olson 2016; Kidder 2003, 261–98).

3. *Case 24:* This kind of case arises for a health system that provides home care and services along the continuum in addition to acute care. Thinking of this kind of case as ultimately involving the application of refined charity care criteria to an unusual circumstance provides a helpful framework and potential guideposts for consideration. In particular, as we saw in case 24, an institution might find obligations to use significant resources to be greater in cases of an ongoing, long-term relationship with a patient.

4. *Case 25:* To whatever extent possible, the ethicist should encourage a deliberative process that considers all the options available and the potential benefits and burdens of each option (Bromage, McLauchlan, and Nightingale 2009). It is very easy to be dismissive of patients who suffer from a

substance use disorder, with the result that all treatments are seen as futile. The ethicist should offer a view of patients who are trying to break an addiction as being simply a variation on the profile of other patients with chronic illnesses. Such a view highlights the fact that patients are often successful in altering their behavioral pattern after repeated attempts rather than on the first attempt. Also, as happened in this case, positive results can last for a period of time but not forever. Nevertheless, when a patient with a chronic illness is treated successfully for two years, such an outcome is generally considered quite worthwhile. Thus, the consultant must work to help the treatment team to see the options in their proper context.

5. *Case 26:* This case is difficult because it involves the behavior of an outside institution over which the receiving institution has no control. The simplest and most important point to keep in mind is that in the short term, the potential receiving hospital needs to be sure that it does not compromise care for a possible patient in an effort to "teach the outside hospital a lesson." Thus, the receiving hospital did well to admit this patient, and it would be ethically correct to do so again under similar circumstances, even though it would have no legal obligation to do so. That is, the patient at issue is not this hospital's patient until it accepts the transfer. But using interinstitutional channels to seek the assistance of administration at the outside hospital seems morally recommended. As the outcome of this case points out, erring on the side of accepting the patient is the correct choice, but it is far better if the patient can be appropriately evaluated at the outside hospital, given that an unnecessary transfer brings its own burdens and risks.

Conceptual Framework:
The Quest for Organizational Ethics,
and the Mission and Stakeholders

What exactly is meant by organizational ethics in health care, and how one "does" such ethics, are not as clear as in the more developed area of bedside clinical ethics. The term "organizational ethics" became widespread in the mid-1990s, when the Joint Commission for the Accreditation of Healthcare Organizations (now formally known as the Joint Commission) added several standards to its review process under the header of organizational ethics. The first issue that it identified was the referral of patients from hospitals to other facilities (e.g., rehabilitation facilities and nursing homes) that were owned by the same corporation as the hospital. The 1990s was an intense period of consolidation in the health care industry, and the word "hospital" commonly was replaced by "health system" as integrated models of care delivery sought to carve out greater shares of their health care markets. The Joint Commission essentially became concerned that patients would be unaware that they had choices with regard to where they would receive their next phase of care and that corporate self-referrals would essentially go unnoticed on this day-to-day level. Thus, the Joint Commission required that each health system have policies and procedures for disclosing its ownership interests in the facilities to which patients were being referred. Although we should be careful about reading too much into history, the original organizational ethics issue in health care was a kind of conflict of interest, and it is related to a mainstream business strategy to control market share. Furthermore, the framework for dealing with the issue borrows a good deal from clinical ethics. That is, the remedy for conflict of interest was essentially seen as disclosure of the conflict and the "informed consent" of the patient.

Despite the elapsing of several decades since these first standards were articulated, it is not clear that anything approximating a field or discipline of organizational ethics has developed. There is no developed literature or identifiable body of knowledge but only a fairly loose collection of topics that tend to be raised under this banner. Some border on clinical issues, such as developing policies and mechanisms for dealing with medical errors or "near misses." Many of the issues seem to involve the allocation of resources—for example, decisions concerning which services should be added or cut, where to invest in new clinics or points of access to the health system, and where to increase or decrease staffing. When someone raises the terminology of organizational ethics in this context, they are usually implicitly or explicitly asking whether one can answer competing claims to resources by drawing on an understanding of the mission of the institution.

Can the mission of an institution be helpful in solving organizational ethics problems? Clearly, the impetus behind this kind of thinking has some historical basis. In particular, most hospital and health systems in the United States are nonprofit corporations. This status means that these corporations' net margins—that is, their profits—are reinvested in the operation of the institution rather than distributed among investors, as happens in a for-profit corporation. A nonprofit corporation is exempt from federal, state, and local taxes. This exemption is given for a reason and should set some expectations for the use of resources, which are often defined in terms of "community benefit."

One way to think about a nonprofit organization is that it received its nonprofit status in order to fulfill a certain mission. A hospital or health system receives this status because it provides an essential service to a particular community. The institution is tax-exempt because the community wishes all funds to be reinvested in providing and extending these services to meet the community's needs. Thus, to some extent, it makes sense to try to resolve organizational questions in accordance with the rationale for the creation of a particular hospital or health system.

Of course, communities change—sometimes quite rapidly in our modern world. Thus, one cannot simply refer to the health care organization's original purpose—for example, a hospital was founded to serve the new wave of Irish immigrants in the early twentieth century, but that purpose and population may no longer be relevant. During this evolution, different persons and groups come to have a stake in the organization. Stakeholders are persons who come to rely on a social arrangement or institution in some identifiable way. Once this reliance is established, altering the arrangement will generally have implications that can be evaluated in ethical terms—that is, with the standard of fairness. This reliance is not necessarily unidirectional but also may mean that the stakeholders contribute to the institution in some way. This confluence of mission that serves stakeholders and comes to embody an organizational culture provides a rich context for ethical decision making (Perry 2014; Boyle et al. 2001).

There are many different kinds of stakeholders in a nonprofit health care organization. First and foremost are the patients the organization serves. Of course, the organization is often a partner or a collaborator with physicians' groups in offering this service. Second, large health care systems employ many people. These employees usually include a variety of health care professionals, such as nurses, therapists, and technicians. Many employees are administrators and administrative staff members, physical plant staff members, and the like. Increasingly, this category also includes physicians, because practice groups are often being merged into health systems. This role as employer can be enormously important, and the hospital or health system may be the major employer in a community. Although this scenario is usually associated with rural communities, even in a large, urban environment—such as Pittsburgh—a health system can be far and away the single largest employer and the region's economic spark plug. It also follows that any number of ancillary businesses may be dependent on an institution, from sandwich shops and retailers to medical waste disposal companies. Third, there are a variety of other kinds of stakeholders in any particular nonprofit health care system. For instance, a sponsoring religious order certainly has a stake in the institution's long-term life and health. Similarly, donors of significant resources have provided funds based on a vision or mission, and thus they hope to see this vision and mission continue to be realized into the future. Also, obviously, the residents of the surrounding community indirectly subsidize the nonprofit organization by forgoing the taxes from the organization that could be gathered if that land were used for a commercial or residential purpose.

This elaboration of the stakeholders' roles is meant to specify the many parties affected by the decisions and policies of a large health care institution, and also to help highlight the complexity of interests that are pertinent to each major decision. Few of these interest groups are silent, even though decision-making processes may not always provide each one with a seat at the table. But a failure to involve significantly affected parties in major decisions also carries its own risks. In particular, decisions made by administrators that have an impact on the medical staff will be very difficult to implement efficiently without the support of physician leaders, even if the physicians are employees. Similarly, a failure to involve other significant stakeholders in decisions can lead to lowered morale and performance, or to a backlash. This situation is clearly to be avoided if one wishes to have a high-quality service orientation.

More than anything else, elaborating the multifarious stakeholders in a nonprofit health system helps us to move beyond the traditional ethics that is tied to a particular physician's virtually unlimited duty to his or her patient, to a thinking that sees sustainability and reconciliation of interests as the goal of ethically appropriate policies. Too often, talk of mission and ethics is seen as unrealistic, and instead fiscal considerations—that is, the margin—are asserted as the only reality. Such a characterization misses the mark. A nonprofit health care institution cannot solve all the community's and society's problems. But it must make a good-faith effort to address the needs of its various stakeholders to the extent possible. Otherwise, the health care system's reason to be ceases to exist. And though the system might not immediately cease to exist along with its mission, it will fail to inspire and to call people into its service. It will likely struggle on an everyday level. At its best, health care is a vocation for those who provide it. Its ethos must be able to call people into its service for it to truly flourish (Lowney 2003).

References and Further Reading

Boyle, Philip J., Edwin R. DuBose, Stephen J. Ellingson, David E. Guinn, and David B. McCurdy. 2001. *Organizational Ethics in Health Care: Principles, Cases, and Practical Solutions*. San Francisco: Jossey-Bass.

Bromage, Daniel I., Duncan J. McLauchlan, and Angus K. Nightingale. 2009. "Do Cardiologists and Cardiac Surgeons Need Ethics? Achieving Happiness for a Drug User with Endocarditis." *Heart* 95, no. 11: 885–87.

Dimaio, Michael J., Tomas A. Salerno, Ron Bernstein, Katia Araujo, Marco Ricci, and Robert M. Sade. 2009. "Ethical Obligation of Surgeons to Noncompliant Patients: Can a Surgeon Refuse to Operate on an Intravenous Drug-Abusing Patient with Recurrent Aortic Valve Prosthesis Infection?" *Annals of Thoracic Surgery* 88, no. 1: 1–8.

Kidder, Tracy. 2003. *Mountains beyond Mountains: The Quest of Paul Farmer, the Man Who Would Cure the World*. New York: Random House.

Kuczewski, Mark G. 2017. "How Medicine May Save the Life of US Immigration Policy: From Clinical and Educational Encounters to Ethical Public Policy." *AMA Journal of Ethics* 19, no. 3: 221–33. http://journalofethics.ama-assn.org/2017/03/peer1-1703.html.

Lee, Esther. 2015. "Health Clinic Refuses to Give Undocumented Immigrant a Kidney Transplant from Her Husband." *ThinkProgress*, June 18. https://thinkprogress.org/health-clinic-refuses-to-give -undocumented-immigrant-a-kidney-transplant-from-her -husband-e873ec27012#.w0hteagkb.

Lowney, Christopher. 2003. *Heroic Leadership: Best Practices from a 450-Year-Old Company That Changed the World.* Chicago: Loyola University Press.

Perry, Frankie. 2014. *The Tracks We Leave: Ethics & Management Dilemmas in Healthcare,* 2nd edition. Chicago: Health Administration Press.

Stone, Geren S., and Kristian R. Olson. 2016. "The Ethics of Medical Volunteerism." *Medical Clinics of North America* 100, no. 2: 237–46.

Wasson, Katherine, and E. David Cook. 2013. "The Common Good and Common Harm." *National Catholic Bioethics Quarterly* 13, no. 4: 617–23.

———. 2014. "The Common Harm in Bioethics and Public Health." *National Catholic Bioethics Quarterly* 14, no. 3: 449–55.

Index

Index

donors: financial, 199; kidney, 29, 30, 169
do-not-resuscitate (DNR) orders: to avoid harm and suffering, 64; decision-making capacity for, 141; family disagreements over, 84; family micromanagement and, 87; patient's wishes and, 14, 60; prehospital, 79–82, 95, 142; surrogate contradiction of, 79–82, 95; unilateral, 106, 107; waiting period and, 56
Dophoff tube (nasogastric tube), 71–72, 73
Drane, James, 44–45
Durable Power of Attorney for Health Care, 51–57, 65, 92, 103

educationally based therapy, 145, 149
elderly patients, decision-making capacity of, 23–27, 40
emancipated minors, 159, 160
emergency care: advance directives in, 15–18, 39–40; as charity care, 170, 180; elderly patients in, 23–24; event model of informed consent and, 45; legal issues for, 172; role of POLST DNR orders in, 79–80; transfer policies and, 187–91, 195
Emergency Medical Treatment and Labor Act, 172
employee-employer relationships, 198–99
endocarditis case studies, 32–36, 40–41, 128–31, 152, 183–86, 194–95
end-of-life decision making, x, 49–111; achieving consensus on, 99–102; classic cases in, 104; conceptual framework for, 97–108; family disagreements and, 83–86, 95; family micromanagement and, 87–90, 95–96; forgoing treatment and, 51–57, 65–70, 91–92, 93; futile medical treatment and, 104–8; informed consent and, 104; patient's wishes

and, 58–64, 92–93; as a process, 100; questionable patient capacity and, 71–74, 93–94; role of POLST DNR orders in, 79–82, 95; substituted judgment and, 103; surrogate decision making and, 75–78, 94, 98, 103–4; values in, 91, 92, 100
end stage renal disease, 167–73, 192–93
equity, health care, xi
ethics consultation services. See clinical ethics case consultations
ethics review committees, 72, 74
event model of informed consent, 45
"everything be done" requests, 29, 58–64, 92–93, 101, 106
experiential interests., 155–56
experimental drug therapy, 137
extraordinary measures, 72
extubation, 60, 76, 77. See also ventilator weaning

fairness, standard of, 198
falls, 23–27
family integrity, 124, 126–27, 132–36, 152, 158, 161
family members: best interests standard and, 13, 157–58; of chronically ill young adults, 137–42, 152–53; coercion and persuasion by, 10–14, 39; communication with, 100–102; cultural values and, 3–9, 39; denial by, 63, 116, 145, 148; disagreements between, 83–86, 95, 137–38; financial power of attorney for, 24, 25, 26; forgoing treatment and, 98–99; heroin addiction in minors and, 128–31, 152; as interpreters, 3–9, 39; micromanagement by, 87–90, 95–96; partnerships with, 150; patient autonomy and, 11–12; patient's mental status and, 29, 30; patient's wishes and, 3–9, 15–18, 39–40, 51–57, 66, 68–69, 92; rights

— 206 —

Index

organizational ethics *(continued)* 194–95; standards for, 196–97; transfer policies and, 187–91, 195

organ transplant case studies. *See* kidney transplant case studies

outpatient treatment, 33, 34

overtreatment, 40. *See also* futile medical treatment

pain, 11, 13, 104, 156–57

palliative care, 14, 20, 151. *See also* comfort care

palliative care consultations, 22, 54, 91, 92, 94, 102

parental authority: best interests of minors and, 121–27, 143–49, 151–52, 153, 155; futile treatment and, 115–20, 151; minors assent and, 159, 160–61; vs. patient's wishes, 137–42, 152–53; religious beliefs and, 115–20, 121–27, 151–52

partnerships, with family members, 150

paternalism, 135, 157–58, 160

patient autonomy: of chronically ill young adults, 160; coercion and, 10–14, 39; competence and, 45; duty of beneficence and, 43; elderly patients and, 25, 26; in emergency settings, 15–18, 39–40; fear of leg amputation and, 19–22, 40; informed consent and, 8, 12, 16, 20–21, 42; interpreter's role and, 3–9, 39; patient's wishes and, 54–55; questionable decision-making capacity and, 73; "sound mind" criteria and, 42–43

patient's wishes: determination of, 99–100; do-not-resuscitate orders and, 14, 60; on forgoing treatment, 66, 68, 93, 97; as the gold standard, 103; as "having everything done," 58–64, 92–93; interpretation of, 93; lack of a Durable Power of Attorney for Health Care and, 51–57, 92; minors and, 118–19, 150–51, 161; vs. parental authority, 137–42, 152–53; vs. professional integrity, 67; surrogate decision making and, 103; values and, 56, 68, 69, 98; variations in, 11, 12, 37–38, 39, 100. *See also* advance directives

payer mix, 170

pediatric hematologists, 125–26

pediatric patients. *See* minors

PEG (percutaneous endoscopic gastrostomy) tube, 71–72, 73, 74

Pentecostal Christians, 168

percutaneous endoscopic gastrostomy (PEG) tube, 71–72, 73, 74

peripherally inserted central catheter (PICC), 28–29, 33, 34, 35–36, 40–41

persistent vegetative state, 84

physiatrists, 144, 147, 149

physical impairments, 156

physician-assisted suicide, 67, 69, 104–5

Physician Order for Life-Sustaining Treatment (POLST), 15–18, 79–82, 92, 95, 103

physician-patient relationship, 9, 45–46, 100–102, 188, 200

physicians: duty of beneficence, 34, 42–43, 135; duty of disclosure, 7, 8–9, 43–44, 197; duty to their patients, 200; as employees, 199; unilateral decision-making by, 92, 107–8

physiological futility, 106–7

PICC (peripherally inserted central catheter), 28–29, 33, 34, 35–36, 40–41

plateaus, in rehabilitation, 145–46, 148

pneumonia, aspiration, 144, 146

POLST (Physician Order for Life-Sustaining Treatment), 15–18, 79–82, 92, 95, 103

Index

postponing death, 106–7

posttransplant care, 168, 169, 170

potentially inappropriate interventions: consensus statement on, 107–8; family micromanagement and, 87–90, 95–96; patient's wishes and, 58–64, 92–93; requests for, 92, 104. *See also* futile medical treatment

power of attorney, financial, 24, 25, 26

practice habits, of health care providers, 99, 102

preferences. *See* patient's wishes

prehospital do-not-resuscitate (DNR) orders, 79–82, 95, 142

privacy, right of, 42

probability of efficacy, 106

process model of informed consent, 45–46

prognosis, information about, 100–102

psychiatric consults, 72, 141, 186

quadriplegic case studies, 143–49, 153, 178–82, 194

quality of life: diminished, 55–56, 119; fear of leg amputation and, 21; forgoing treatment and, 107; futile medical treatment and, 106; probability of, 62, 76, 168

Quinlan, Karen Ann, 99, 104

rationing care, 184

recovery, partial, 55–56

referral relationships, 187–91, 195, 196–97

refusal of treatment. *See* treatment refusal

rehabilitation ethics, 143–49, 153

rehabilitation programs, 153, 185, 186

reimbursement, for home health care, 178–79

religious beliefs, 115–20, 121–27, 151–52

resource allocation, xi; administrators and, 192; charity care criteria and, 178–82, 194; margins and, 171, 179, 192, 193, 197–98, 200; medical mission patients and, 174–77; organizational ethics and, 197; substance use disorder and, 183, 184; undocumented immigrants and, 167–73, 192–93

restraints, 29, 31

resuscitation. *See* cardiopulmonary resuscitation

risk(s): competence and, 44–45; informed consent and, 8, 44–45, 97; transfer policies and, 189, 190, 191, 195

scarcity, 28, 184, 185

SCD (sickle cell disease) case study, 121–27, 151–52

Schiavo, Terri, 99

Schloendorf, Mary, 42

Schloendorf case, 42

second opinions, 120

self-determination: of chronically ill young adults, 137–42, 152–53, 159; forgoing treatment and, 105; informed consent and, 107; right of, 42, 43

septal defect case study, 174–77, 194

sickle cell disease (SCD) case study, 121–27, 151–52

skill builder cases, xii–xiii, xiv; care for undocumented immigrants, 167–73, 192–93; forgoing life-sustaining treatment, 51–57, 92; futile treatment and religious beliefs of minors, 115–20, 151; patient's wishes and futile treatment, 58–64, 92–93; truth telling and culture, 3–9, 39

skilled nursing facilities, 35–36, 76

social media, 168

About the Authors

Mark G. Kuczewski, PhD, is the Father Michael I. English, SJ, Professor of Medical Ethics, the director of the Neiswanger Institute for Bioethics and Health Policy, and the chair of the Department of Medical Education in the Stritch School of Medicine—all at Loyola University Chicago.

Rosa Lynn B. Pinkus, PhD, served as professor of medicine/neurosurgery, associate director for the Center of Bioethics and Health Law, and director of the Consortium Ethics Program, University of Pittsburgh. She retired in December 2013 and currently teaches a graduate bioethics course for the Department of Bioengineering, University of Pittsburgh.

Katherine Wasson, PhD, MPH, is an associate professor and bioethicist at the Neiswanger Institute for Bioethics and Health Policy at Loyola University Chicago Stritch School of Medicine.